Melanoma

Editors

KIMBERLY M. BROWN
CELIA CHAO

SURGICAL CLINICS
OF NORTH AMERICA

www.surgical.theclinics.com

Consulting Editor
RONALD F. MARTIN

October 2014 • Volume 94 • Number 5

ELSEVIER

1600 John F. Kennedy Boulevard • Suite 1800 • Philadelphia, Pennsylvania, 19103-2899

http://www.surgical.theclinics.com

SURGICAL CLINICS OF NORTH AMERICA Volume 94, Number 5
October 2014 ISSN 0039–6109, ISBN-13: 978-0-323-32682-7

Editor: John Vassallo, j.vassallo@elsevier.com
Developmental Editor: Yonah Korngold

Surgical Clinics of North America (ISSN 0039–6109) is published bimonthly by Elsevier Inc., 360 Park Avenue South, New York, NY 10010-1710. Months of publication are February, April, June, August, October, and December. Business and Editorial Offices: 1600 John F. Kennedy Blvd., Suite 1800, Philadelphia, PA 19103-2899. Periodicals postage paid at New York, NY and additional mailing offices. Subscription prices are $370.00 per year for US individuals, $627.00 per year for US institutions, $180.00 per year for US students and residents, $455.00 per year for Canadian individuals, $793.00 per year for Canadian institutions, $510.00 for international individuals, $793.00 per year for international institutions and $250.00 per year for Canadian and foreign students/residents. To receive student/resident rate, orders must be accompanied by name of affiliated institution, date of term, and the *signature* of program/ residency coordinator on institution letterhead. Orders will be billed at individual rate until proof of status is received. Foreign air speed delivery is included in all *Clinics* subscription prices. All prices are subject to change without notice. POSTMASTER: Send address changes to *Surgical Clinics*, Elsevier Health Sciences Division, Subscription Customer Service, 3251 Riverport Lane, Maryland Heights, MO 63043. **Customer Service (orders, claims, online, change of address): Telephone: 1-800-654-2452 (U.S. and Canada); 314-447-8871 (outside U.S. and Canada). Fax: 314-447-8029. E-mail: journalscustomerservice-usa@elsevier.com (for print support); journalsonline support-usa@elsevier.com (for online support)**.

Reprints. For copies of 100 or more, of articles in this publication, please contact the Commercial Reprints Department, Elsevier Inc., 360 Park Avenue South, New York, New York 10010-1710. Tel. 212-633-3874, Fax: 212-633-3820, E-mail: reprints@elsevier.com.

The Surgical Clinics of North America is also published in Spanish by McGraw-Hill Interamericana Editores S.A., P.O. Box 5-237 06500 Mexico D.F. Mexico; and in Portuguese by Interlivros Edicoes Ltda., Rua Comandante Coelho 1085, CEP 21250, Rio de Janeiro, Brazil; and in Greek by Paschalidis Medical Publications, Athens Greece.

The Surgical Clinics of North America is covered in *MEDLINE/PubMed (Index Medicus)*, *EMBASE/Excerpta Medica*, *Current Contents/Clinical Medicine*, *Current Contents/Life Sciences*, *Science Citation Index*, and *ISI/BIOMED*.

Contributors

CONSULTING EDITOR

RONALD F. MARTIN, MD, FACS
Staff Surgeon, Department of Surgery, Marshfield Clinic, Marshfield, Wisconsin; Clinical Associate Professor, University of Wisconsin School of Medicine and Public Health, Madison, Wisconsin; Colonel, Medical Corps, United States Army Reserve

EDITORS

KIMBERLY M. BROWN, MD
Assistant Professor, Department of Surgery, University of Texas Medical Branch, Galveston, Texas

CELIA CHAO, MD, FACS
Associate Professor, Department of Surgery, University of Texas Medical Branch, Galveston, Texas

AUTHORS

ANDREA M. ABBOTT, MD, MS
Department of Cutaneous Oncology, Moffitt Cancer Center, Tampa, Florida

SAÏD C. AZOURY, MD
Halsted Surgery Resident, Department of Surgery, The Johns Hopkins Hospital, Johns Hopkins Medicine, Baltimore, Maryland

CELIA CHAO, MD, FACS
Associate Professor, Department of Surgery, University of Texas Medical Branch, Galveston, Texas

STEVEN L. CHEN, MD, MBA
Associate Professor, Department of General Oncologic Surgery, City of Hope National Medical Center, Duarte, California

JERRY CHERIYAN, MD, MRCS
Department of General Surgery, Marshfield Clinic, Marshfield, Wisconsin

ERIC G. DAVIS, MD
Assistant Professor, The Hiram C. Polk Jr, Department of Surgery, University of Louisville School of Medicine, Louisville, Kentucky

MARK B. FARIES, MD
Director, Donald L. Morton Melanoma Research Program, John Wayne Cancer Institute, Santa Monica, California

GEOFFREY T. GIBNEY, MD
Assistant Member, Department of Cutaneous Oncology, Moffitt Cancer Center; Assistant Professor, Department of Oncologic Sciences, USF Morsani College of Medicine, Tampa, Florida

MARK A. HEALY, MD
Resident, Department of Surgery, University of Michigan, Ann Arbor, Michigan

JOHN M. KANE III, MD
Chief, Melanoma-Sarcoma Service, Department of Surgical Oncology, Roswell Park Cancer Institute, Buffalo, New York

RONDI M. KAUFFMANN, MD, MPH
Department of General Oncologic Surgery, City of Hope National Medical Center, Duarte, California

BRENT KELLY, MD
Associate Professor, Department of Dermatology, University of Texas Medical Branch, Galveston, Texas

CHARLES W. KIMBROUGH, MD
The Hiram C. Polk, Jr, Department of Surgery, University of Louisville School of Medicine, Louisville, Kentucky

JULIE R. LANGE, MD, ScM
Associate Professor, Department of Surgery, The Johns Hopkins Hospital, Johns Hopkins Medicine, Baltimore, Maryland

DELPHINE J. LEE, MD, PhD
Director of Carolyn Dirks and Brett Dougherty Laboratory for Cancer Research; Director of Department of Translational Immunology, John Wayne Cancer Institute, Santa Monica, California

KELLY M. McMASTERS, MD, PhD
Ben A. Reid Sr, MD, Professor and Chairman, The Hiram C. Polk Jr, Department of Surgery, University of Louisville School of Medicine, Louisville, Kentucky

JANE L. MESSINA, MD
Dermatopathologist, Departments of Anatomic Pathology and Cutaneous Oncology, Moffitt Cancer Center; Professor, Departments of Pathology & Cell Biology and Dermatology, USF Morsani College of Medicine, Tampa, Florida

AMY A. MRAZEK, MD
General Surgery Resident, Department of Surgery, University of Texas Medical Branch, Galveston, Texas

JACQUELINE OXENBERG, DO
Department of Surgical Oncology, Roswell Park Cancer Institute, Buffalo, New York

JUNKO OZAO-CHOY, MD
Department of Surgery, Harbor-UCLA Medical Center, Torrance, California

VERNON K. SONDAK, MD
Chair, Department of Cutaneous Oncology, Moffitt Cancer Center; Professor of Surgery, Departments of Oncologic Sciences and Surgery, USF Morsani College of Medicine, Tampa, Florida

JONATHAN STUBBLEFIELD, BS
School of Medicine, University of Texas Medical Branch, Galveston, Texas

ANDREW URQUHART, MD, FACS
Department of Otolaryngology/Head and Neck Surgery, Marshfield Clinic, Marshfield, Wisconsin

IRIS H. WEI, MD
Resident, Department of Surgery, University of Michigan, Ann Arbor, Michigan

JESSICA WERNBERG, MD, FACS
Adjunct Clinical Assistant Professor, Department of General Surgery/Surgical Oncology, Marshfield Clinic, Marshfield, Wisconsin

SANDRA L. WONG, MD, MS
Associate Professor, Department of Surgery, University of Michigan, Ann Arbor, Michigan

JONATHAN S. ZAGER, MD, FACS
Director of Regional Therapies; Associate Member; Department of Cutaneous Oncology, Moffitt Cancer Center, Tampa, Florida

Contents

> The incidence of melanoma has increased over the past several decades. Despite improved case mortality, overall deaths from melanoma have increased because of the large increase in incidence. Although we have a better understanding of the pathogenesis of melanoma and improved early diagnostic capabilities, the burden of disease and societal costs remain high. This article provides an update on the epidemiology of cutaneous melanoma worldwide and the common risk factors including heritable and modifiable risks, emphasizing the importance of education, early detection, and prevention in reducing the disease burden.

> Melanoma continues to be one of the fastest growing cancers in terms of incidence. The workup of melanoma focuses on risk factors based on the visual aspects of a skin lesion. Risk factors including sun exposure increase the risk of melanoma. Staging is based on depth of invasion, mitotic rate, and spread into lymph nodes and other sites. Once diagnosed, wide excision is indicated for the primary lesion, and sentinel node biopsy for all but the thinnest of melanomas. Routine imaging workup for most thinner melanomas should be minimized, and is questionable in the asymptomatic patients even with thicker melanomas.

> Although melanoma represents less than 5% of all skin cancers, it is responsible for the bulk of skin cancer–related deaths. Nevertheless, despite this aggressive reputation, most patients with cutaneous melanoma will be surgically cured of their disease. Early detection allows for curative resection, and 5-year survival for all stages of melanoma is 91%. This review outlines the surgical treatment of melanoma, including principles of wide local excision and management of the regional lymph nodes.

> The number of melanoma survivors in the United States continues to steadily increase 2.6% per year, while death rates have remained stable

over time. Although controversy exists regarding optimal surveillance strategies, recommendations for clinical monitoring are based on tumor stage, tumor phenotype, likelihood of recurrence, prognosis, risk factors, psychosocial impact of disease, and patient well-being. Management guidelines for recurrent disease depend on the type of recurrence: local, satellite/in-transit, regional, or distant metastasis. This article is a current review of the literature concerning melanoma survivorship.

In-transit disease is defined as any dermal or subcutaneous metastases that arise between the primary melanoma but not beyond the draining regional nodal basin. Patients who develop in-transit disease are at further risk to develop additional locoregional and distant disease. Treatment must be individualized and take into consideration the extent of disease, tumor characteristics, and patient characteristics including age, comorbidities, previous therapies, and site of recurrence. Surgery, regional perfusions and intralesional injections all play a role in management options. These patients should be discussed and managed by a multidisciplinary team whenever possible.

Cancer vaccines were one of the earliest forms of immunotherapy to be investigated. Past attempts to vaccinate against cancer, including melanoma, have mixed results, showing the complexity of what was believed to be a simple concept. However, several recent successes and the combination of improved knowledge of tumor immunology and the advent of new immunomodulators make vaccination a promising strategy for the future.

Although melanoma was historically thought to be radiation resistant, there are limited data to support the use of adjuvant radiation therapy for certain situations at increased risk for locoregional recurrence. High-risk primary tumor features include thickness, ulceration, certain anatomic locations, satellitosis, desmoplastic/neurotropic features, and head and neck mucosal and anorectal melanoma. Lentigo maligna can be effectively treated with either adjuvant or definitive radiation therapy. Some retrospective and prospective randomized studies support the use of adjuvant radiation to improve regional control after lymph node dissection for high-risk nodal metastatic disease. Consensus on the optimal radiation doses and fractionation is lacking.

The management of unresectable metastatic melanoma has dramatically improved in recent years. Surgeons need to familiarize themselves with new drugs and the biology behind them, and ongoing clinical trials and new drugs in development for adjuvant therapy and treatment of metastatic disease.

SURGICAL CLINICS
OF NORTH AMERICA

Foreword

Melanoma

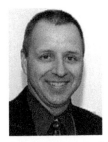

Ronald F. Martin, MD, FACS
Consulting Editor

We are all products of our mentors to some degree. As a student, I relish this. As I mentor, it sometimes terrifies me. The reason for each is the same: we remember vividly those things we were told as students by our mentors and take and keep them to heart—right or wrong. Fortunately for me, my mentors told me things that have held up well over time and in many respects they were prescient if not visionary. For my students, I'll let them write about it after they get out of therapy. One of my mentors, Dr Walter Goldfarb, influenced me more than any other. I could write a whole book rather than a foreword (and probably should someday) about the lessons he gave us. Walter's most amazing gift was not only knowing what seemed to be everything but also being able to weave it seamlessly into almost any clinical encounter in a memorable and almost always hysterical way. In particular, he always reminded me that to really understand things one has to be patient and to read and think a lot and for a long time. He more than anyone showed me how "great new ideas" were almost always recycled ideas. Not to say that the recycled ideas are always bad ones—some ideas have to wait for their time. He knew where and when the ideas came from originally. When they came around refreshed, he usually knew if they were really "new and improved" or just recycled. Walter unfailingly knew the genuine article when he saw it.

Another mentor who deeply influenced my thinking was another genius named Dr Blake Cady. I didn't get to work with Blake as closely or for as long as I would have liked, but thankfully, even a short time spent with Blake was enlightening. Blake could effortlessly quote chapter and verse of just about anything written. In a meeting, in a clinical setting, out for a walk, or over a drink—no matter where, he managed to educate while having a good time.

As a rule, I really don't care for people wistfully and pithily recalling their training heroes in presentations (or forewords) under the guise that other people should feel strongly toward their "heroes." This is no exception. I don't bring them up because I wish for you to see them as I do but because each of them made something clear to me that we should all know. One day, Walter and I were discussing melanoma and he spoke the now time-remembered quote, "Ronnie, deep down inside we're all superficial!" And he meant this on many levels as was appropriate. This lesson didn't just refer to the depth of invasion of the tumor in the patient but in the depth or shallowness of some people who bring us the "truth."

Blake's quotes are also numerous and memorable. Perhaps my favorite though is on his commentary on a multinational melanoma study that failed to address its stated hypothesis but was claiming great discovery and import anyway. After an incredibly post-hoc subset analysis, the paper claimed significance for a small subset of a small subset of patients. Blake's immortal retort from the microphone at that time of presentation was, "[This study] shows that if one tortures the data long enough, they will confess to something!"

So what does any of this have to do with melanoma? Well, as it turns out, melanoma is a bit interesting in many respects. The incidence is up but the mortality is down. Increased awareness makes it more popular to the layperson than some other less conspicuous diseases. In an era of declining reimbursement, it provides low time-intensive, low morbidity procedures that are still well reimbursed. Perhaps, though, more importantly than all the above is that it takes a very long time to find out what kind of impact changes in management have—perhaps more than a career's worth of time. That last bit is a double-edged sword. While it makes it hard to challenge or be challenged successfully in real time, it also makes it hard to find out whether our ideas were right or not in time to publish them. It is pretty common to see this response when someone does challenge a conclusion: "We are still collecting this data and while I can say that it absolutely supports what I have already said we won't be able to release that information formally for a few years."

Time! Time! You can't make it go faster and you can't slow it down. We are all victims of our impatience. We all suffer from the 24-hour news cycle. Our news media struggle to be fastest, not the most accurate. Our stock traders covet communications capabilities that will let them trade milliseconds ahead of a competitor. Our learners want bulleted information that "just gives the answer they need" without any of that context fluff. Our texting-addicted culture would eschew most vowels and consonants that are not phonetically required. Yet time is the great equalizer. It's not for sale at any price.

In the field of human inquiry, one must sometimes be patient. One must occasionally set the wheels in motion and accept that someone else will reap the credit for deciphering the conclusions. The more indolent the disease, the narrower the treatment difference, and the longer we must wait to see if we were right. When it comes to melanoma, we need to design trials and live with the results they yield rather than manipulate trials part way through because "we have spent so much time already we have to get something out of this." We need to be more reflective, and we need to drink deeper from the well of knowledge. We need to be less superficial.

Of course, you will never know where to begin if you don't know what we have looked through so far. To that end, Drs Brown and Chao and their colleagues have given us a sound foundation on which to build. I urge the reader not only to read the articles but also to pull out the references and dig deeply. You have time. You will be rewarded. In particular, I owe Dr Brown a deep debt of thanks for the many times, including this effort, when she has taken on a project at my request despite her own demands.

Despite the seemingly increasing desire to learn just enough in the least amount of time, when it comes to melanoma, we need to be less superficial and more reflective. We need to torture the data less and be more skeptical and inquisitive about our results. We need to make sure that what we do is not just statistically significant but also clinically significant. And when we feel pressured and challenged about why we don't know all the answers faster, perhaps, ironically, we just need to have a thicker skin.

Ronald F. Martin, MD, FACS
Department of Surgery
Marshfield Clinic
1000 North Oak Avenue
Marshfield, WI 54449, USA

E-mail address:
martin.ronald@marshfieldclinic.org

Preface

Melanoma

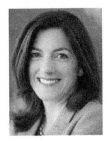 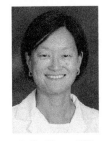

Kimberly M. Brown, MD   Celia Chao, MD
Editors

In the last issue of *Surgical Clinics of North America* devoted to melanoma, a double issue published in February and April 2003, Dr Stanley P.L. Leong, Guest Editor, remarked on the new advances in melanoma diagnosis and treatment that had occurred since the 1996 issue devoted to cutaneous melanoma. As guest editors for this issue, it is fair and accurate to once again marvel on how much our understanding and approach to this disease have evolved in the last decade. We are privileged to have collaborated with world-class authors and experts on melanoma.

Although the incidence of melanoma is increasing worldwide, recent overall five-year survival for patients with melanoma exceeds 90% in the United States. As described by Dr Lange and colleagues, melanoma is being approached as a public health problem, which integrates basic and clinical science with education efforts around prevention and early detection right where the rubber meets the road—including schools, primary care office, and dermatology clinics. In addition to established risk factors such as UV exposure, we now have more sophisticated genetic markers of increased risk, which may help focus early detection resources.

Drs Kauffmann and McMasters review the evidence-based approach for the staging workup and surgical treatment, respectively, of melanoma. The recent maturity of several significant clinical trials has better informed decision-making around sentinel lymph node biopsy and lymph node dissection across the spectrum of disease burden. In addition, there have been advancements in understanding of the complex interactions between the host immune system and the tumor, which have shaped the locoregional approaches to melanoma, new systemic and targeted therapies, the role of radiation in melanoma treatment, and the future directions of melanoma vaccines. These topics are eloquently presented by Drs Zager, Sondak, Kane, and Faries, respectively.

Advancements in surgical, locoregional, systemic, and targeted therapy have widened options for the treatment of patients with advanced, metastatic melanoma, which may result now in prolonged quality and quantity of life. The multidisciplinary approach to patients with stage IV melanoma is described by Dr Wong and colleagues,

Surg Clin N Am 94 (2014) xv–xvi
http://dx.doi.org/10.1016/j.suc.2014.07.012
0039-6109/14/$ – see front matter © 2014 Published by Elsevier Inc.

surgical.theclinics.com

including the integration of prognostic tumor biology data into the decision-making for surgical and other therapies, as well as the use of tumor-specific mutations as targets for new biologic agents. Melanoma survivorship has become even more important given the increased survival rates for patients in recent years. Drs Chao and Mrazek review the evidence-based approach to survivorship, including surveillance and management of recurrence.

Melanoma is not just a cutaneous disease, and Dr Sondak provides an excellent description of the approach to unusual melanoma presentations, such as ocular melanoma, melanoma of unknown primary, mucosal melanoma, and melanoma in childhood. In addition, Drs Urquhart and Wernberg discuss the unique features and treatment approaches associated with head and neck presentations of melanoma, and Dr Kelly and colleagues review melanoma presenting in non-Caucasian patients.

Optimal medical management of patients with melanoma in the twenty-first century requires a multidisciplinary approach, including, but not limited to, general surgeons, surgical oncologists, head and neck surgeons, medical oncologists, dermatologists, primary care physicians, and radiation therapists. We are grateful to our colleagues for their invaluable contributions to this issue. We also wish to express our gratitude to Eileen Figueroa in the Department of Surgery at the University of Texas Medical Branch and the editorial staff at Elsevier for their assistance.

Kimberly M. Brown, MD
Department of Surgery
University of Texas Medical Branch
301 University Boulevard
Galveston, TX 77555, USA

Celia Chao, MD
Department of Surgery
University of Texas Medical Branch
301 University Boulevard
Galveston, TX 77555, USA

E-mail addresses:
km3brown@utmb.edu (K.M. Brown)
cechao@utmb.edu (C. Chao)

Epidemiology, Risk Factors, Prevention, and Early Detection of Melanoma

Saïd C. Azoury, MD, Julie R. Lange, MD, ScM*

KEYWORDS

• Melanoma • Epidemiology • Risk factors • Screening • Early detection • Prevention

KEY POINTS

- The incidence of melanoma has increased worldwide over the past several decades.
- Melanoma is the fifth most common cancer in men and the seventh most common cancer in women in the United States. Overall survival has improved, with a 5-year survival of nearly 91% in the United States.
- Risk factors in the development of melanoma include environmental exposures and host factors. Ultraviolet light has been implicated in the pathogenesis of melanoma.
- Educational programs should be encouraged to help increase public awareness. Clinicians and patients should be familiar with the clinical ABCDEs to promote early detection and diagnosis.
- Worldwide, better strategies for prevention and early detection are needed.

INTRODUCTION

Although melanoma accounts for less than 5% of all skin cancers diagnosed, the disease burden of melanoma is significant, with an estimated 50,000 deaths annually worldwide.[1] Melanoma is the fifth most common cancer in men and seventh most common cancer in women in the United States.[2] Compared with other common malignancies, melanoma has a relatively high 5-year survival. In the last 20 years, overall 5-year survival has increased in the United States, from approximately 82% to greater than 91% in 2013.[3] In addition to the life-threatening potential of melanoma, the disease has a large economic impact. Over the past several decades, there has been a steady increase in the incidence of melanoma around the world. Increased detection of early-stage lesions and increased recreational exposure to ultraviolet (UV) radiation

Disclosures: None.
Department of Surgery, The Johns Hopkins Hospital, Johns Hopkins Medicine, 600 North Wolfe Street, Blalock 610, Baltimore, MD 21287, USA
* Corresponding author.
E-mail address: jlange@jhmi.edu

Surg Clin N Am 94 (2014) 945–962
http://dx.doi.org/10.1016/j.suc.2014.07.013
0039-6109/14/$ – see front matter © 2014 Elsevier Inc. All rights reserved.

surgical.theclinics.com

may both have contributed to this increase in incidence.[4] Fortunately, survival in this same period has steadily improved, likely a result of earlier diagnosis.[3]

Strides in basic science and clinical research have led to the development of newer therapies for patients with advanced disease, including immunotherapy and targeted therapies. Efforts should also focus on improving awareness among both the public and health care providers to help facilitate early detection and prevention. Although the association of harmful environmental exposures (eg, sunlight) and melanoma is familiar, equally important risk factors include family history and personal medical history. The advent of modern technologies has given insight into many potential genetic associations. Today greater efforts are being made in education, early detection, and prevention. Optimal control of melanoma as a public health burden requires a team approach and the coordinated effort of basic scientists, primary care physicians, dermatologists, surgeons, oncologists, and other health care professionals.

EPIDEMIOLOGY AND IMPACT
Global Incidence

Globally there has been a steady increase in melanoma incidence over the past 50 years, with nearly 200,000 new cases diagnosed annually.[1,2,5] The incidence of melanoma in Caucasians is inversely related to one's distance from the equator.[6] New Zealand and Australia have the highest incidence of melanoma worldwide.[7] In 2002 in Queensland, Australia, there were 82.1 cases of invasive melanoma per 100,000 per year for men and 55.3 per 100,000 per year for women.[8] In New Zealand in 1999, the crude annual incidence for invasive melanoma was 77.7 per 100,000 per year.[9] In Europe, the highest incidence in males is seen in Germany, Norway, and Switzerland while Denmark, Iceland, Norway, and Switzerland have the highest incidence in females.[10]

In the United States melanoma incidence has increased, with annual-age standardized increases estimated at 2% to 4%.[2,3,11] In 1992, the incidence was 18.2 per 100,000; by 2004, it had increased to 26.3 per 100,000.[4] In the United States in 2014, it is predicted that an estimated 76,100 patients will be diagnosed with invasive melanoma, with 9710 melanoma-related deaths.[2] Melanoma accounts for nearly 4.6% of all reported newly diagnosed malignancies, but this may not include some thin superficial and in situ melanomas that may be underreported to cancer registries.[2,12,13]

Economic Impact

Although few studies have examined the impact of melanoma on the economy, the cost to the American health care system is significant. The annual cost of treating newly diagnosed melanoma has been estimated to be anywhere from $563 million to more than $1 billion in the United States.[14] In addition, the cost of treating a single stage I patient is roughly 40-fold less than the cost of treating one stage III or stage IV patient.[14] With early-stage disease most of the treatment and follow-up can be done on an outpatient basis. However, in cases of advanced disease the cost of management and related care is exceedingly high. Together, stage III and IV disease account for 90% of the total annual direct costs.[14]

Demographics and Trends

Race

Some differences in the incidence and anatomic distribution patterns of melanoma are related to race. Melanoma occurs far more commonly in Caucasians than in persons of other races.[15] Overall, Caucasians, African Americans, Asians/Pacific Islanders, and American Indians/Alaskan Natives account for 95%, 0.5%, 0.3%, and 0.2% of the cases reported to the Surveillance, Epidemiology and End Results Program

(SEER) in the United States, respectively.[16] Non-Caucasians tend to present at a more advanced stage at diagnosis and have a lower overall 5-year survival compared with Caucasians.[15,16] Possible reasons for differences in presentation include a decreased suspicion among patients and clinicians for skin lesions, less noticeable anatomic sites such as the soles of the feet or digits, and limited access to educational and health care resources.

A study using data from 38 population-based cancer registries in the United States analyzed trends for various racial groups.[16] Overall, the median age of diagnosis was 59 to 63 years of age for African American and Caucasian patients alike and 52 to 56 years of age in the other racial groups including Hispanics, American Indians, and Asians.[16] Distant metastasis at presentation was observed in fewer than 5% of Caucasian patients compared with 7% to 13% of the other groups. Most of the Caucasian patients (63%) were diagnosed with thin melanomas (≤1.0 mm in thickness). In African Americans, acral lentiginous melanoma was the most common histologic type, whereas superficial spreading melanoma was most common among the other racial and ethnic groups.[16] The incidence of acral lentiginous melanoma was highest overall in Hispanic and African American patients (**Fig. 1**).[16] The most common anatomic site among Caucasians and American Indians is the trunk, whereas in African Americans and Asian Pacific Islanders the most common sites are the lower limbs and hip.[16]

Gender

Overall, melanoma is more common in men than in women, and survival is worse in men.[2,17] The American Cancer Society estimates that in 2014 approximately 43,890 men and 32,210 women in the United States will be diagnosed with melanoma.[2] In a recent Minnesota review, from 1970 to 2009 there was an 8-fold increase in incidence in young women aged 18 to 39 years, with only a 4-fold increase in young men.[18] The overall melanoma incidence ratio in men compared with women in the United States is age dependent.[2] Whereas the probability of developing melanoma in women younger than 49 years is higher than in men, after this age men experience a sharp increase in incidence and have an overall higher likelihood of developing this malignancy.[2] In males, the most common anatomic sites are the head and neck, whereas in females the extremities and the torso/trunk are most commonly affected.

Age

Melanoma in young persons Age is well recognized as an important factor in the epidemiology of melanoma. Though the disease is far more common in adults, it

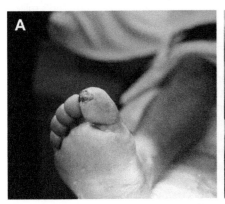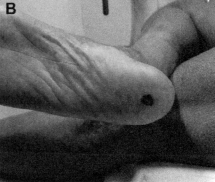

Fig. 1. Acral lentiginous melanoma on the great toe (*A*) and sole of the foot (*B*).

can be found in children, accounting for 1% to 4% of all melanomas.[19–21] The incidence of melanoma in pediatric patients is reported to have increased by 46% from 1973 to 2001.[19] A study using patients from the National Cancer Data Base reported a male predominance in patients aged 1 to 9 years, most notable in the youngest patients.[21] Primary tumors were found to be thicker in children younger than 15 years compared with older teenagers and young adults.[21] Survival in children is related to the extent of disease. Although the incidence in children and young adults is increasing, melanoma case mortality in children appears to be decreasing.[21,22]

Melanoma in older persons Older patients have poorer survival in comparison with younger patients.[20] A recent report from the expanded American Joint Committee on Cancer database demonstrated that patients older than 70 years have melanomas with more aggressive prognostic features compared with other age groups.[22] The primary lesions found in this age group tend to be increased in thickness, more ulcerated, and have higher mitotic rates.[22] In addition, most melanomas in the elderly were noted to arise in the scalp, head, and neck, with fewer diagnosed on the trunk and lower extremities. Elderly patients also have a higher incidence of acral lentiginous melanomas, desmoplastic melanomas, and lesions that have more spindle cell features.[22]

Overall incidence and mortality trends for men and women are similar; however, among those aged 65 years and older, the increase in incidence has been higher in men (5-fold in men compared with 3-fold in women).[23] Between 1969 and 1999, the mortality rates of melanoma increased from 2 to 3 per 100,000.[23] This increase is mostly attributed to the significant increase observed in the geriatric population. In fact, in this time period in persons aged 20 to 44 years, there was a decrease in mortality by 39% (from 1.3 to 0.8 per 100,000) in women and by 29% (from 1.7 to 1.2 per 100,000) in men.[23] In men and women aged 45 to 64 years, mortality rates increased by 66% (from 3.8 to 6.3 per 100,000) and 19% (from 2.6 to 3.1 per 100,000), respectively.[23] Mortality rates increased by 157% (from 7.5 to 19.3 per 100,000) in men older than 65 years (more than 3-fold greater than the trend observed in women older than 65 years).[23]

RISK FACTORS

Melanoma causation and risk association is complex, with genetic and environmental factors affecting individual risk (**Fig. 2**). As noted earlier, Caucasian race, male sex, and older age are well-recognized factors associated with an increased risk of developing melanoma. In general, risk factors for melanoma can be categorized as related to either personal host factors or environmental exposures.

Host Factors

Personal cancer history

- Having a history of melanoma or nonmelanoma skin cancer significantly increases one's risk for developing cutaneous melanoma. Regardless of the type of skin cancer, studies have demonstrated nearly a 3-fold relative risk of acquiring melanoma in these individuals.[24–28]
- Melanoma risk has been associated with a personal history of other adult malignancies, including brain, breast, prostate, and other cancers.[25–28]
- The future risk of cutaneous melanoma was analyzed in the Childhood Cancer Survivor Study. Individuals with a childhood history of sarcoma, lymphoma, leukemia, and or central nervous system tumors had up to a 2.5-fold increased risk of developing melanoma in the future.[29]

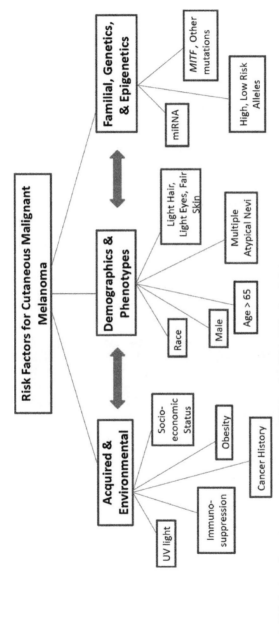

Fig. 2. Risk factors for cutaneous melanoma. miRNA, microRNA; UV, ultraviolet.

Predisposing skin lesions

- Among Caucasians, the number of benign melanocytic nevi and atypical nevi influence melanoma risk.[30] Risk is higher with increased numbers of both common and atypical nevi (**Fig. 3**).
- Giant congenital nevi are associated with a greatly increased risk of melanoma.[31] The cumulative 5-year risk of cutaneous melanoma in these patients has been estimated at 5.7%.[32]

Select phenotypes: hair and eye color

Two high-risk groups for melanoma are fair-skinned individuals with red or blond hair with many freckles, and individuals with darker hair and skin with a high melanocytic nevi count.[33] Patients who have a darker complexion are considered to be less photosensitive than individuals with red hair, lighter skin, and blue eyes, and have lower personal risk of melanoma.[33] With regard to hair color, red hair implies the greatest risk followed by blonde and light brown hair. Similarly, lighter colored eyes (blue or hazel) are associated with a greater risk than are dark brown eyes.[33]

Family history and genetics

- Individuals with a positive family history of melanoma have a relative risk of 1.74 compared with those with negative family history.[23] Approximately 10% of patients with melanoma have a positive family history.[4]
- Mutation in the *MITF* gene predisposes to both familial and sporadic melanoma.[34]
- Germline mutations in *CDKN2A* and *CDK4* have been identified in familial melanoma.[35–38]
- The red-hair phenotype has been associated with Melanocortin-1 receptor (*MC1R*), which has further been linked to cutaneous melanoma.[39,40]

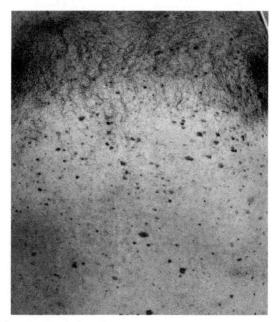

Fig. 3. A man with many atypical nevi.

- Individuals with dysplastic nevus syndrome (also known as familial BK mole syndrome, familial atypical multiple-mole melanoma syndrome, and familial melanoma syndrome) have a reported cumulative lifetime risk of up to 100%.[41,42]
- *RB1* is a high-penetrance allele for melanoma.[43]
- A mutation in BRCA-associated protein 1 (BAP1) has been found in families with multiple generations of cutaneous melanoma.[44] Similarly, *BRCA2* gene mutation has been associated with increased melanoma risk.[45]
- Records from Genome-Wide Association Studies have identified single-nucleotide polymorphisms that are associated with melanoma, and certain phenotypic characteristics of melanoma.[46]
- There is an increased risk of melanoma in patients with xeroderma pigmentosum, a rare autosomal recessive disease associated with a severe deficiency in nucleotide excision repair.[47] The exact risk association has been difficult to quantify.[47]

Epigenetics

MicroRNAs are short ($\sim$22 nucleotides) noncoding RNAs that can regulate gene expression posttranscriptionally, and their dysregulation may have implications in melanoma development.[48] The mechanism and impact of these findings have not been fully elucidated.

Exposures

Ultraviolet light

UV light is the best known and most investigated exogenous risk factor for developing melanoma.[49–58] The exact causal relationship is complex. Both intermittent, intense UV light exposure (eg, sunburn history) and chronic, cumulative amount of sun exposure play a role in the pathogenesis of melanoma.[49]

Mechanism Recent data have provided biological evidence for UV-induced melanoma carcinogenesis. Significant mutations in *STK19*, *RAC1*, and *PPP6C* resulting from C>T transitions have been identified as a result of direct UVB-mediated damage.[52] In addition, the p53 tumor suppressor gene mutation has been reported in many cases of melanoma, and UV radiation has been hypothesized to play a role in its mutagenesis.[50,52] In mouse models, interferon-γ has been shown to promote UVB-induced melanocyte activation, survival, and immunoevasion.[53] Similarly, repetitive UV exposure may promote angiogenesis and melanoma metastasis.[57]

Exposure and anatomic location Melanoma risk at different anatomic sites is associated with varying patterns and amounts of UV exposure.[51] Individuals with melanomas of the head and neck often have had high levels of occupational sun exposure, and therefore develop lesions more frequently on these sun-exposed body parts.[51,58] Head and neck melanomas are also associated with other sequelae of sun exposure, including presence of solar keratoses and a history of treatment of solar skin lesions.[58] Conversely, melanomas of the same histologic type occurring on the trunk (ie, a site of less sun exposure) tend to occur in people with lower levels of sun exposure and fewer solar keratoses.[58,59]

Artificial tanning Tanning-bed usage has been linked to the development of melanoma.[60] The International Agency for Research on Cancer has concluded that there is a direct causal relation.[61] Artificial tanning has gained popularity over the past several decades. Tanning beds are advertised as having a similar ratio of UVA to UVB as sunlight; however, some artificial units emit much higher amounts of UV radiation.[62] It has been estimated that 70% of the estimated 28 million persons in the

United States who engage in artificial tanning are women aged 16 to 49 years.[63,64] Similarly, the Centers for Disease Control and Prevention and the National Cancer Institute reported higher rates of indoor tanning among women, whites, and adults aged 18 to 25 years.[65]

In 2007 The World Health Organization (WHO) International Agency for Research on Cancer showed that individuals whose first use of a tanning bed was before 35 years of age had up to a 75% greater risk of developing melanoma in comparison with those individuals who have never used tanning beds.[62] Moreover, the risk of developing melanoma in indoor tanners seems to be related to the frequency of exposure, as the risk has been shown to increase with the number of sunbed tanning sessions.[60] Analyses performed in Iceland demonstrated a sharp increase in the incidence of melanoma among women younger than 50 years in the years following an increase in the popularity of artificial tanning; the incidence among women younger than 50 subsequently decreased after implementation of interventions to discourage artificial tanning.[66]

Immunosuppression

As with other malignancies, the increase in incidence and poorer prognosis of melanoma with increasing age may be due, in part, to accumulation of cellular damage over time and decreased host defense and immune surveillance.[67–71]

There is a higher incidence of cutaneous malignant melanoma, up to 3- to 4-fold, in patients after organ transplantation, presumed to be related to medical immunosuppression.[72] The interval to diagnosis of melanoma after organ transplantation typically ranges from nearly 5 to 11 years, and the mean age at diagnosis is 54 years.[73] Cutaneous melanoma tends to be more advanced at presentation in organ transplant patients. In addition, when compared with cases in nontransplanted patients in the SEER database, a poorer prognosis of melanoma has been observed in patients with a history of transplantation regardless of tumor thickness.[74] Transplant recipients with lesions thicker than 1.51 mm had significantly decreased overall survival compared with nontransplanted patients with melanoma of similar stage.[74]

Socioeconomic status

The incidence of malignant melanoma has increased across all socioeconomic groups.[4] However, individuals in the lowest socioeconomic quintiles present at more advanced stages, and the group with the lowest socioeconomic status has shown the steepest rise in the incidence of thick tumors (>4 mm).[4] In addition, superficial spreading melanomas are less common in individuals of lower socioeconomic status, whereas aggressive nodular and acral lentiginous melanomas are common in this group.[75]

In a study looking at melanoma cases in the California Cancer Registry records, 27% of Medicaid enrollees were found to have nodal or distant disease at diagnosis, whereas only 9% of non-Medicaid enrollees had similarly advanced disease.[76] In the United Kingdom, it has been shown that people from more socially deprived districts are more reluctant to seek advice for a suspicious lesion.[77] Similarly, a review of insurance status and race using the US National Cancer Database noted a significantly higher likelihood of uninsured patients being diagnosed with advanced-stage melanoma in comparison with privately insured patients; the odds ratios for advanced-staged melanomas were 2.3 for uninsured patients and 3.3 for Medicaid-insured patients.[78] Older individuals covered by Medicare residing in areas of lower socioeconomic status have a lower survival rate and a greater likelihood of having a higher stage at presentation compared with older individuals residing in areas of higher socioeconomic status.[79]

Individuals with low socioeconomic status have poorer access to health care in the United States.[4] Implementation of education and prevention strategies targeted at high-risk subgroups of low socioeconomic status promises to be an important strategy in a public health approach to melanoma control.

Other Factors

Other possible associations or factors influencing melanoma risk have been less well studied, and some reports have presented conflicting conclusions:

- One study on immunosuppressive therapy, reviewing long-term use of tumor necrosis factor α for longer than 120 days in patients with inflammatory bowel disease, reported an odds ratio of 3.93 in comparison with those without long-term use.[80]
- A potential protective effect of nonsteroidal anti-inflammatory drug use with regard to developing melanoma has been described.[81]
- There have been no conclusive data to support a role of pregnancy or hormones in the risk of melanoma carcinogenesis.[82]
- One meta-analysis noted that there was an increased risk of melanoma in overweight and obese males, although no obvious association was observed in women.[83]
- Evidence for the association between levels of vitamin D and melanoma is inconclusive.[84]
- Several studies have noted an association between Parkinson's disease and an increased incidence of melanoma.[85–87]

PREVENTION AND EARLY DETECTION
Prevention

Avoiding excess UV radiation exposure is to date the best prevention measure to decrease an individual's risk of developing melanoma. Randomized controlled trials have demonstrated that primary care counseling interventions may help decrease indoor tanning and increase sun-protective behaviors.[88] Better adherence to screening recommendations and sun-protection strategies is associated with female gender, sun-sensitive phenotype (eg, red hair, fair skin), greater perceived benefits of sun protection, physician's recommendation for screening, and greater perceived risk of skin cancer.[89] Examples of protective measures include avoiding artificial tanning and excessive sun exposure, and wearing sunscreen and protective clothing. One particular study, begun in 1992, randomized 1621 participants to either discretionary or daily application of sunscreen to the head and neck.[90] This study reported a nonsignificant trend toward a protective effect of daily application of sunscreen against cutaneous melanoma.[90]

Children, adolescents, and young adults are important target age groups for prevention efforts. The US Preventive Services Task Force (USPSTF) recommends advising fair-skinned young persons, aged 10 to 24 years, to minimize UV radiation exposure.[91,92] The WHO and the International Commission on Non-Ionizing Radiation Protection recommend against the use of artificial tanning devices in individuals younger than 18 years and those with high-risk phenotypes (eg, presence of premalignant or malignant skin lesions).[93,94] In the United States, California and Vermont were among the first to ban the use of tanning beds for youths younger than 18 years. Most US states have some artificial tanning restrictions in place for minors.[95] The American Cancer Society has recommended against the use of tanning beds in general across all age groups.[96]

Early Detection

Education

Even with the advances made in melanoma diagnosis over the last several decades, many lesions are missed at earlier stages, this being a result of both patient and provider factors.[97] Melanomas may be missed at anatomic sites that the patient cannot easily see. Moreover, melanomas are diagnosed at more advanced stages in low-risk patients (eg, non-Caucasians or those with low sun exposure), perhaps a result of lower suspicion and decreased awareness in these patients and their physicians.[97] Hence, although high-risk groups, by definition, are more likely to have melanoma, education to promote early detection should also include lower-risk groups.[97]

Efforts should be made to promote education and outreach programs. The American Cancer Society recommends monthly self-examinations of skin.[96,98] In general, both patients and clinicians should be well familiar with the A, B, C, D, and E signs of melanoma.[98,99]

- *A*symmetry: one half does not match the other (**Figs. 4** and **5**)
- *B*orders: irregular, not well defined; can be notched, scalloped, or angulated (see **Figs. 4** and **5**)
- *C*olor: often dark brown or black; but can be variegated with some lighter brown, red, bluish, or grayish areas (see **Figs. 4** and **5**; **Fig. 6**)
- *D*iameter: large, increasing, greater than 6 mm (see **Fig. 5**; **Fig. 7**)
- *E*volving: changes over time including growth, change in color, or new symptoms such as itching or bleeding

Timely recognition is critical to improving outcomes. Although most melanomas have one or more of the ABCDE findings, some may not display any of the ABCDEs. Some lesions are amelanotic and may not display any of these signs, potentially delaying a diagnosis. For example, diagnostic delay is common with the subtype desmoplastic melanoma, which is often amelanotic and can be sometimes be mistaken for a scar or other benign skin lesion.[100]

For those individuals at high risk of developing melanoma, particularly those with many atypical nevi, total-body photography is sometimes used for surveillance and diagnosis.[4] Epiluminescence microscopy, or dermoscopy, allows magnification levels up to 10-fold and rapid in vivo observation of skin lesions with a hand-held device.[101] Dermoscopy allows a skilled examiner to observe the coloration and microstructures of the epidermis, the dermoepidermal junction, and the papillary dermis. In the hands of a skilled dermatologist, dermoscopy can result in greater sensitivity and specificity

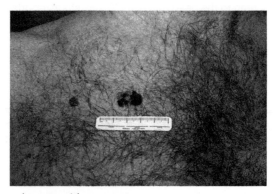

Fig. 4. Cutaneous melanoma with asymmetry.

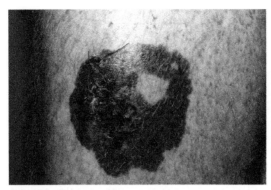

Fig. 5. Cutaneous melanoma with irregular borders.

in the evaluation of pigmented lesions. Newer, computer-assisted diagnostic instruments are under investigation.[101]

Early detection

When melanoma is diagnosed early and properly treated, outcomes and survival are favorable. In 2009, it was estimated that to demonstrate a significant impact on mortality, upward of $40 million would be needed to screen a population of 350,000 Americans older than 45 years, with a 4-year intervention period and an 8-year follow-up interval.[102] One cost-effectiveness model from 2007, however, did show that a melanoma screening program involving a once per lifetime screening test was indeed cost-effective when compared with other current cancer screening programs.[103]

The initial detection of melanomas is most often by the patients themselves. However, physicians who are skilled and well aware of melanoma presentation are able to diagnose melanoma at earlier stages.[97] Physician detection is associated with melanomas thinner than those detected by patients or family members.[97,104,105] A partial skin examination can easily be performed during the usual heart and lung physical examination.[102] Some have suggested that primary care physicians and medical students are not adequately trained in skin examination.[102] Physicians who had more information sources such as pamphlets and brochures were more likely to fully examine their patients.[106] Physicians are more likely to examine patients if the patients themselves raise concerns about new skin lesions or request a skin evaluation.[107] The literature has shown that access to and use of a dermatologist correlates with better melanoma survival in general.[102]

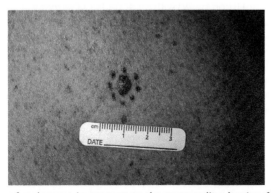

Fig. 6. Darker hue of melanoma in contrast to the surrounding benign freckles.

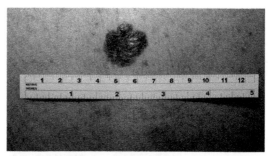

Fig. 7. Note the large diameter of this melanoma at diagnosis.

The increase in the incidence of melanoma in the geriatric population, particularly in older white men, has been well documented. In 2000, however, the Institute of Medicine concluded that owing to insufficient direct evidence, conclusions could not be made regarding the effectiveness of a clinical screening program of asymptomatic Medicare beneficiaries.[108] More recently, the USPSTF concluded that there is insufficient evidence to recommend total-body skin examinations for routine screening of cutaneous melanoma, basal cell cancer, or squamous cell cancer.[109] However, the benefits of early detection and treatment as part of usual medical care were emphasized, and patients and clinicians were advised to continue to closely monitor any changes in skin examinations and to be aware of common signs of skin cancer.[108] As the incidence and proportion of thicker melanomas in the older population continues to increase, more effective efforts in early detection should be developed.

Recently, greater efforts have been made to establish direct evidence for the benefits of routine screening for melanoma. The American Academy of Dermatology has provided free screening programs and melanoma/skin cancer education since 1985.[110] Initial data demonstrated that 33% of screened individuals reported a change in a mole, 8% reported a family history of melanoma, 3% reported a personal history of melanoma, and 65% had at least 1 identifiable risk factor. Nearly 80% of these individuals did not have a regular dermatologist, and 60% had never had their skin checked by a doctor.[110]

Some evidence supports the idea that early detection through screening can have an impact on disease stage and mortality. In Germany, a screening program of more than 360,000 residents used both dermatologists and nondermatologists. In the screened area of Germany, melanoma incidence increased by 30% relative to the rest of the country. However, melanoma-related mortality decreased by 7.4% per year (nearly 50% overall) compared with other parts of Germany and with Denmark.[111] In Queensland, Australia, screening was associated with a 38% greater likelihood of being diagnosed with a thinner melanoma ($\leq$0.75 mm).[112] Whole-body clinical skin examination performed before diagnosis was associated with a 14% reduced risk of being diagnosed with a melanoma greater than 0.75 mm in thickness.[112] A separate study from Queensland, Australia observed that older people, men, and those who had not been screened by a health care provider in the 3 years before the study were more likely to have nodular tumors of greater thickness.[113]

SUMMARY

Decreasing the morbidity and mortality of cutaneous melanoma requires a multidisciplinary approach involving primary care specialists in addition to dermatologists, oncologists, surgeons, and other health care providers in the overall management.

Equally important, patients should seek care as soon as possible for any concerning skin changes. Skin cancer education programs should continue to be strongly encouraged for all individuals at low and high risk alike, to increase awareness in the general population. Unfortunately, prevention and early detection programs lack a uniform approach worldwide, and targeting high-risk groups remains a challenge. Encouraging a consensus on these initiatives can reduce the morbidity and mortality of melanoma and lessen the cost of melanoma in health care systems.

REFERENCES

1. Ferlay J, Shin HR, Bray F, et al. Estimates of worldwide burden of cancer in 2008: GLOBOCAN 2008. Int J Cancer 2010;127(12):2893–917.
2. Siegel R, Ma J, Zou Z, et al. Cancer statistics. CA Cancer J Clin 2014;64:9–29.
3. Available at: http://www.seer.cancer.gov/statfacts. Accessed November 5, 2013.
4. Linos E, Swetter SM, Cockburn MG, et al. Increasing burden of melanoma in the United States. J Invest Dermatol 2009;129(7):1666–74.
5. Erdmann F, Lortet-Tieulent J, Schüz J, et al. International trends in the incidence of malignant melanoma 1953-2008—are recent generations at higher or lower risk? Int J Cancer 2013;132(2):385–400.
6. Armstrong BK. Epidemiology of malignant melanoma: intermittent or total accumulated exposure to the sun? J Dermatol Surg Oncol 1988;14(8):835–49.
7. Sneyd MJ, Cox B. A comparison of trends in melanoma mortality in New Zealand and Australia: the two countries with the highest melanoma incidence and mortality in the world. BMC Cancer 2013;13(1):372.
8. Coory M, Baade P, Aitken J, et al. Trends for in situ and invasive melanoma in Queensland, Australia, 1982-2002. Cancer Causes Control 2006;17(1):21–7.
9. Jones WO, Harman CR, Ng AK, et al. Incidence of malignant melanoma in Auckland, New Zealand: highest rates in the world. World J Surg 1999;23(7):732–5.
10. Karim-Kos HE, de Vries E, Soerjomataram I, et al. Recent trends of cancer in Europe: a combined approach of incidence, survival and mortality for 17 cancer sites since the 1990s. Eur J Cancer 2008;44:1345–89.
11. Geller AC, Clapp RW, Sober AJ, et al. Melanoma epidemic: an analysis of six decades of data from the Connecticut Tumor Registry. J Clin Oncol 2013;31(33):4172–8.
12. Cockburn M, Swetter SM, Peng D, et al. Melanoma under-reporting: why does it happen, how big is the problem, and how do we fix it? J Am Acad Dermatol 2008;59(6):1081.
13. Hall HI, Jamison P, Fulton JP, et al. Reporting cutaneous melanoma to cancer registries in the United States. J Am Acad Dermatol 2004;49(4):624–30.
14. Tsao H, Rogers GS, Sober AJ. An estimate of the annual direct cost of treating cutaneous melanoma. J Am Acad Dermatol 1998;38:669–80.
15. Cormier JN, Xing Y, Ding M. Ethnic differences among patients with cutaneous melanoma. Arch Intern Med 2006;166(17):1907–14.
16. Wu XC, Eide MJ, King J, et al. Racial and ethnic variations in incidence and survival of cutaneous melanoma in the United States 1999-2006. J Am Acad Dermatol 2011;65(5):1–13.
17. Hohnheiser AM, Gefeller O, Göhl J. Malignant melanoma of the skin: long-term follow-up and time to first recurrence. World J Surg 2011;35(3):580–9.
18. Reed KB, Brewer JD, Lohse CM, et al. Increasing incidence of melanoma among young adults: an epidemiological study in Olmsted County, Minnesota. Mayo Clin Proc 2012;87(4):328–34.

19. Strouse JJ, Fears TR, Tucker MA, et al. Pediatric melanoma: risk factor and survival analysis of the Surveillance, Epidemiology and End Results database. J Clin Oncol 2005;23(21):4735–41.

20. Averbook BJ, Lee SJ, Delman KA, et al. Pediatric melanoma: analysis of an international registry. Cancer 2013;119(22):4012–9.

21. Lange JR, Palis BE, Chang DC, et al. Melanoma in children and teenagers: an analysis of patients from the National Cancer Data Base. J Clin Oncol 2007;25: 1363–8.

22. Balch CM, Soong S, Gershenwald JE, et al. Age as a prognostic factor in patients with localized melanoma and regional metastases. Ann Surg Oncol 2013;20:3961–8.

23. Geller AC, Miller DR, Annas GD, et al. Melanoma incidence and mortality among US whites, 1969-1999. JAMA 2002;288:1719–20.

24. Rhodes AR, Weinstock MA, Fitzpatrick TB, et al. Risk factors for cutaneous melanoma. A practical method of recognizing predisposed individuals. JAMA 1987; 258:3146–54.

25. Tucker MA, Boice JD Jr, Hoffman DA. Second cancer following cutaneous melanoma and cancers of the brain, thyroid, connective tissue, bone, and eye in Connecticut, 1935-82. Natl Cancer Inst Monogr 1985;68:161–89.

26. Abern MR, Tsivian M, Coogan CL, et al. Characteristics of patients diagnosed with both melanoma and renal cell cancer. Cancer Causes Control 2013; 24(11):1925–33.

27. Levi F, Te VC, Randimbison L, et al. Cancer risk in women with previous breast cancer. Ann Oncol 2003;14(1):71–3.

28. Li WQ, Qureshi AA, Ma J, et al. Personal history of prostate cancer and increased risk of incident melanoma in the United States. J Clin Oncol 2013; 31(35):4394–9.

29. Pappo AS, Armstrong GT, Liu W, et al. Melanoma as a subsequent neoplasm in adult survivors of childhood cancer: a report from the Childhood Cancer Survivor Study. Pediatr Blood Cancer 2013;60:461–6.

30. Gandini S, Sera F, Cattaruzza MS, et al. Meta-analysis of risk factors for cutaneous melanoma: I. Common and atypical naevi. Eur J Cancer 2005;41:28–44.

31. Swerdlow AJ, English JSC, Qiao Z. The risk of melanoma in patients with congenital nevi: a cohort study. J Am Acad Dermatol 1995;32(4):595–9.

32. Egan CL, Oliveria SA, Elenitsas R, et al. Cutaneous melanoma risk and phenotypic changes in large congenital nevi: a follow-up study of 46 patients. J Am Acad Dermatol 1998;39(6):923–32.

33. Gandini S, Sera F, Cattaruzza MS, et al. Meta-analysis of risk factors for cutaneous melanoma: III. Family history, actinic damage and phenotypic factors. Eur J Cancer 2005;41:2041–59.

34. Yokoyama S, Woods SL, Boyle GM, et al. A novel recurrent mutation in MITF predisposes to familial and sporadic melanoma. Nature 2011;480:99–103.

35. Goldstein AM, Chan M, Harland M, et al. Features associated with germline CDKN2A mutations: a GenoMEL study of melanoma-prone families from three continents. J Med Genet 2007;44(2):99–106.

36. Zuo L, Weger J, Yang Q, et al. Germline mutations in the p16INK4a binding domain of CDK4 in familial melanoma. Nat Genet 1996;12(1):97–9.

37. Haluska FG, Hodi FS. Molecular genetics of familial cutaneous melanoma. J Clin Oncol 1998;16(2):670–82.

38. Curtin JA, Fridlyand J, Kageshita T, et al. Distinct sets of genetic alterations in melanoma. N Engl J Med 2005;353:2135–47.

39. Valverde P, Healy E, Jackson I, et al. Variants of the melanocyte-stimulating hormone receptor gene are associated with red hair and fair skin in humans. Nat Genet 1995;11(3):328–30.

40. Ralmondi S, Sera F, Gandini S, et al. MC1R variants, melanoma and red hair color phenotype: a meta-analysis. Int J Cancer 2008;122:2753–60.

41. Rigel DS, Rivers JK, Friedman RJ, et al. Risk gradient for malignant melanoma in individuals with dysplastic naevi. Lancet 1988;1(8581):352–3.

42. Green MH, Clark WH Jr, Tucker MA, et al. High risk of malignant melanoma in melanoma-prone families with dysplastic nevi. Ann Intern Med 1985;102(4):458–65.

43. Fletcher O, Easton D, Anderson K, et al. Lifetime risks of common cancers among retinoblastoma survivors. J Natl Cancer Inst 2004;96(5):357–63.

44. Njauw CN, Kim I, Piris A, et al. Germline BAP1 inactivation is preferentially associated with metastatic ocular melanoma and cutaneous-ocular melanoma families. PLoS One 2012;7(4):335295.

45. Debniak T, Scott RJ, Górski B, et al. Common variants of DNA repair genes and malignant melanoma. Eur J Cancer 2008;44(1):110–4.

46. Gudbjartsson DF, Sulem P, Stacey SN, et al. ASIP and TYR pigmentation variants associate with cutaneous melanoma and basal cell carcinoma. Nat Genet 2008;40(7):886–91.

47. Paszkowska-Szczur K, Scott RJ, Serrano-Fernandez P, et al. Xeroderma pigmentosum genes and melanoma risk. Int J Cancer 2013;133(5):1094–100.

48. Bennett PE, Bemis L, Norris DA, et al. miR in melanoma development: miRNAs and acquired hallmarks of cancer in melanoma. Physiol Genomics 2013;45:1049–59.

49. Gandini S, Sera F, Cattaruzza MS, et al. Meta-analysis of risk factors for cutaneous melanoma: II. Sun exposure. Eur J Cancer 2005;41:45–60.

50. Jhappan C, Noonan FP, Merlino G. Ultraviolet radiation and cutaneous malignant melanoma. Oncogene 2003;22(20):3099–112.

51. Chang YM, Barrett JH, Bishop DT, et al. Sun exposure and melanoma risk at different latitudes: a pooled analysis of 5700 cases and 7216 controls. Int J Epidemiol 2009;38(3):814–30.

52. Hodis E, Watson IR, Kryukov GV, et al. A landscape of driver mutations in melanoma. Cell 2012;150:251–63.

53. Zaidi MR, Davis S, Noonan FP, et al. Interferon-γ links ultraviolet radiation to melanomagenesis in mice. Nature 2011;469(7331):548–53.

54. Berger MF, Hodis E, Hefferman TP, et al. Melanoma genome sequencing reveals frequent PREX2 mutations. Nature 2012;485:502–6.

55. Noonan FP, Recio JA, Takayama H, et al. Neonatal sunburn and melanoma in mice. Nature 2001;413(6853):271–2.

56. Gilchrest BA, Eller MS, Geller AC, et al. The pathogenesis of melanoma induced by ultraviolet radiation. N Engl J Med 1999;340(17):1341–8.

57. Bald T, Quast T, Landsberg J, et al. Ultraviolet-radiation-induced inflammation promotes angiotropism and metastasis in melanoma. Nature 2014;507(7490):109–13.

58. Whiteman DC, Watt P, Purdue DM, et al. Melanocytic nevi, solar keratosis, and divergent pathways to cutaneous melanoma. J Natl Cancer Inst 2003;95:806–12.

59. Caini S, Gandini S, Sera F, et al. Meta-analysis of risk factors for cutaneous melanoma according to anatomical site and clinico-pathological variant. Eur J Cancer 2009;45:3054–63.

60. Boniol M, Autier P, Boyle P, et al. Cutaneous melanoma attributable to sunbed use: systematic review and meta-analysis. BMJ 2012;345:1–12.

61. Gandini S, Autier P, Boniol M. Reviews on sun exposure and artificial light and melanoma. Prog Biophys Mol Biol 2011;107:362–6.
62. IARC Working Group on Artificial UV light and Skin Cancer. The association of use of sunbeds with cutaneous malignant melanoma and other skin cancers: a systematic review. Int J Cancer 2007;120:1116–22.
63. Kwon HT, Mayer JA, Walker KK, et al. Promotion of frequent tanning sessions by indoor tanning facilities: two studies. J Am Acad Dermatol 2002;46:700–5.
64. Swerdlow AJ, Weinstock MA. Do tanning lamps cause melanoma? An epidemiologic assessment. J Am Acad Dermatol 1998;38:89–99.
65. Centers for Disease Control and Prevention (CDC). Use of indoor tanning devices by adults—United States, 2010. MMWR Morb Mortal Wkly Rep 2012; 61(18):323–6.
66. Héry C, Tryggvadottir L, Sigurdsson T, et al. A melanoma epidemic in Iceland: possible influence of sunbed use. Am J Epidemiol 2010;172(7):762–7.
67. Balch CM, Soong SJ, Gershenwald JE, et al. Prognostic factors analysis of 17,600 melanoma patients: validation of the American Joint Committee on Cancer melanoma staging system. J Clin Oncol 2001;19(6):3622–34.
68. Finkel T, Serrano M, Blasco MA. The common biology of cancer and ageing. Nature 2007;448:767–74.
69. Curtis HJ. Biological mechanisms underlying the aging process. Science 1963; 141(3582):686–94.
70. Lange JR, Kang S, Balch CM. Melanoma in the older patient: measuring frailty as an index of survival. Ann Surg Oncol 2011;18(12):3531–2.
71. Tsai S, Balch C, Lange J. Epidemiology and treatment of melanoma in elderly patients. Nat Rev Clin Oncol 2010;7(3):148–52.
72. Lindelof B, Sigurgeirsson B, Gabel H, et al. Incidence of skin cancer in 5356 patients following organ transplantation. Br J Dermatol 2000;143:513–9.
73. DePry JL, Reed KB, Cook-Norris RH, et al. Iatrogenic immunosuppression and cutaneous malignancy. Clin Dermatol 2011;29:602–13.
74. Brewer JD, Christenson LJ, Weaver AL, et al. Malignant melanoma in solid transplant recipients. Arch Dermatol 2011;147(7):790–6.
75. Pollitt RA, Clarke CA, Swetter SM, et al. The expanding melanoma burden in California Hispanics: importance of socioeconomic distribution, histologic subtype, and anatomic location. Cancer 2011;117(1):152–61.
76. Pollitt RA, Clarke CA, Shema SJ, et al. California Medicaid enrollment and melanoma stage at diagnosis: a population-based study. Am J Prev Med 2008; 35(1):7–13.
77. Eiser JR, Pendry L, Greaves CJ, et al. Is targeted early detection for melanoma feasible? Self assessments of risk and attitudes to screening. J Med Screen 2000;7:199–202.
78. Halpern MT, Ward EM, Pavluck AL, et al. Association of insurance status and ethnicity with cancer stage at diagnosis for 12 cancer sites: a retrospective analysis. Lancet Oncol 2008;9(3):222–31.
79. Reyes-Ortiz CA, Goodwin JS, Freeman JL, et al. Socioeconomic status and survival in older patients with melanoma. J Am Geriatr Soc 2006;l54:1758–64.
80. Long MD, Martin CF, Pipkin CA, et al. Risk of melanoma and nonmelanoma skin cancer among patients with inflammatory bowel disease. Gastroenterology 2012;143:390–9.
81. Johannesdottir SA, Chang ET, Mehnert F, et al. Nonsteroidal anti-inflammatory drugs and the risk of skin cancer: a population-based case-control study. Cancer 2012;118:4768–76.

82. Gandini S, Iodice S, Koomen E, et al. Hormonal and reproductive factors in relation to melanoma in women: current review and meta-analysis. Eur J Cancer 2011;47: 2607–17.

83. Sergentanis TN, Antoniadis AG, Gogas HJ, et al. Obesity and risk of malignant melanoma: a meta-analysis of cohort and case-control studies. Eur J Cancer 2013;49:642–57.

84. Asgari MM, Maruti SS, Kushi LH, et al. A cohort study of vitamin D intake and melanoma risk. J Invest Dermatol 2009;129(7):1675–80.

85. Bajaj A, Driver JA, Schernhammer ES. Parkinson's disease and cancer risk: a systemic review and meta-analysis. Cancer Causes Control 2010;21:697–707.

86. Fiala KH, Whetteckey J, Manyam BV. Malignant melanoma and levodopa in Parkinson's disease: causality or coincidence? Parkinsonism Relat Disord 2003;9: 321–7.

87. Liu R, Gao X, Lu Y, et al. Meta-analysis of the relationship between Parkinson disease and melanoma. Neurology 2011;76:2002–9.

88. Available at: www.cancer.org/cancer/news/study-links-tanning-bed-use-to-increased-risk-of-melanoma. Accessed November 25, 2013.

89. Kasparian NA, Mcloone JK, Meiser B. Skin cancer-related prevention and screening behaviors: a review of the literature. J Behav Med 2009;32(5):406–28.

90. Green AC, Williams GM, Logan V, et al. Reduced melanoma after regular sunscreen use: randomized trial follow-up. J Clin Oncol 2011;29(3):257–63.

91. Moyer VA, U.S. Preventive Services Task Force. Behavioral counseling to prevent skin cancer: U.S. Preventive Services Task Force recommendation statement. Ann Intern Med 2012;157(1):59–65.

92. Lin JS, Eder M, Weinmann S. Behavioral counseling to prevent skin cancer: a systematic review for the U.S. Preventive Services Task Force. Ann Intern Med 2011;154(3):190–201.

93. International Commission on Non-Ionizing Radiation Protection (ICNIRP). Health issues of ultraviolet tanning appliances used for cosmetic purposes. Health Phys 2003;84(1):119–27.

94. Available at: http://www.who.int/uv/publications/en/sunbeds.pdf?ua=1. Accessed March 5, 2014.

95. Geller AC, Balk SJ, Fisher DE. Stemming the tanning bed epidemic: time for action. J Natl Compr Canc Netw 2012;10(10):1311–4.

96. Available at: http://www.cancer.org/cancer/cancercauses/sunanduvexposure/skincancerpreventionandearlydetection/skin-cancer-prevention-and-early-detection-skin-exams. Accessed March 25, 2014.

97. Schwartz JL, Wang TS, Hamilton TA, et al. Thin primary cutaneous melanomas: associated detection patterns, lesion characteristics, and patient characteristics. Cancer 2002;95(7):1562–8.

98. Abbasi NR, Shaw HM, Rigel DS, et al. Early diagnosis of cutaneous melanoma: revisiting the ABCD criteria. JAMA 2004;292(22):2771–6.

99. Friedman RJ, Rigel DS, Kopf AW. Early detection of malignant melanoma: the role of physician examination and self-examination of the skin. CA Cancer J Clin 1985;35:130–51.

100. Wood BA. Desmoplastic melanoma: recent advances and persisting challenges. Pathology 2013;45(5):453–63.

101. Rigel DS, Russak J, Friedman R. The evolution of melanoma diagnosis: 25 years beyond the ABCDs. CA Cancer J Clin 2010;60:301–16.

102. Geller AC. Educational and screening campaigns to reduce deaths from melanoma. Hematol Oncol Clin North Am 2009;23:515–27.

103. Losina E, Walensky RP, Geller A, et al. Visual screening for malignant melanoma: a cost-effectiveness analysis. Arch Dermatol 2007;143(1):21–8.
104. Epstein DS, Lange JR, Gruber SB, et al. Is physician detection association with thinner melanomas? JAMA 1999;281(7):640–3.
105. Brady MS, Oliveria SA, Christos PJ, et al. Patterns of detection in patients with cutaneous melanoma. Cancer 2000;89(2):342–7.
106. Geller AC, O'Riordan DL, Oliveria SA, et al. Overcoming obstacles to skin cancer examinations and prevention counseling for high-risk patients: results of a national survey of primary care physicians. J Am Board Fam Pract 2004; 17(6):416–23.
107. Geller AC, Swetter SM, Oliveria S, et al. Reducing mortality in individuals at high risk for advanced melanoma through education and screening. J Am Acad Dermatol 2011;65(5):1–69.
108. Institute of Medicine. Extending Medicare coverage for prevention and other services. Washington, DC: National Academy Press; 2000.
109. U.S. Preventive Services Task Force. Screening for skin cancer: U.S. Preventive Services Task Force recommendation statement. Ann Intern Med 2009;150(3): 188–93.
110. Geller AC, Zhang Z, Sober AJ, et al. The first 15 years of the American Academy of Dermatology skin cancer screening programs: 1985-1999. J Am Acad Dermatol 2003;48(1):34–41.
111. Katalinic A, Waldmann A, Weinstock MA, et al. Does skin cancer screening save lives? An observational study comparing trends in melanoma mortality in regions with and without screening. Cancer 2012;118:5395–402.
112. Aitken JF, Elwood M, Baade PD, et al. Clinical whole-body skin examination reduces the incidence of thick melanomas. Int J Cancer 2010;126:450–8.
113. Geller AC, Elwood M, Swetter SM, et al. Factors related to the presentation of thin and thick nodular melanoma from a population-based cancer registry in Queensland Australia. Cancer 2009;115:1318–27.

Workup and Staging of Malignant Melanoma

Rondi M. Kauffmann, MD, MPH, Steven L. Chen, MD, MBA*

KEYWORDS

- Melanoma • Skin neoplasms • Melanoma workup • Melanoma staging

KEY POINTS

- Melanoma is the fifth most common cancer in the United States, and its incidence is increasing.
- Skin lesions with asymmetry, irregular borders, heterogeneous coloration, increasing diameter, or changes over time should be investigated for possible melanoma.
- Pathologic reports after skin biopsy should include important prognostic factors, including histologic subtype, Breslow depth, dermal mitotic rate, and presence of lymphocytic invasion, ulceration, or regression.
- Sentinel lymph node biopsy is important for staging, prognosis, and treatment planning.
- Radiologic assessment for metastases should be performed routinely only in those with symptomatic stage III melanoma.

INTRODUCTION

Melanoma is the fifth most common cancer in the United States, with an estimated 76,100 new cases and 9710 deaths in 2014.[1,2] The incidence has steadily increased over the past 4 decades, with an average increase of 2.6% per year for each of the last 10 years, making it one of the most rapidly rising cancers in terms of incidence.[3] Although the largest number of melanoma cases occurs in individuals aged 55 to 64 years, is it the most common cancer in adults aged 25 to 29 years, and the second most common cancer in adolescents.[4]

Risk factors for melanoma include history of blistering sunburn (particularly at a young age), personal history of melanoma, family history, immune suppression, presence of multiple atypical moles, chronic sun or tanning bed exposure, or genetic syndromes, such as Wiskott-Aldrich syndrome or *xeroderma pigmentosa*. In addition, individuals with red or blond hair, fair complexion, or light eyes are at increased lifetime

The authors have nothing to disclose.
Department of General Oncologic Surgery, City of Hope National Medical Center, 1500 East Duarte Road, Duarte, CA 91010-3000, USA
* Corresponding author.
E-mail address: schenmd@gmail.com

Surg Clin N Am 94 (2014) 963–972
http://dx.doi.org/10.1016/j.suc.2014.07.001
0039-6109/14/$ – see front matter © 2014 Elsevier Inc. All rights reserved.

risk for melanoma.[4] Melanoma frequently occurs in existing moles, and early signs of melanoma are described by the mnemonic "ABCDE" (**Fig. 1**).[5]

PRINCIPLES OF BIOPSY

The first step to accurately staging a patient with suspected melanoma is a complete history and physical examination, including complete examination of the entirety of the skin and all draining lymph node basins. Lesions suspicious for melanoma should be biopsied, taking care to obtain sufficient tissue to allow for accurate assessment of the

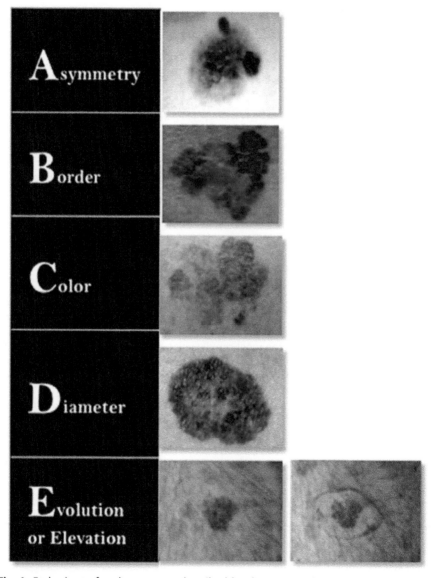

Fig. 1. Early signs of melanoma are described by the mnemonic "ABCDE". (*Courtesy of* Jae Jung, MD, Department of Dermatology, City of Hope Medical Center, Duarte, CA; and Dr Lynn Cornelius, Washington University, St Louis, MO.)

depth of invasion, if present, which in general should be a full-thickness biopsy. Small lesions that are not in cosmetically sensitive locations are amenable to excisional biopsy. An elliptical incision should be oriented to allow for wide excision of the lesion should it reveal melanoma, which is usually along skin lines, or the longitudinal axis of the extremity. Particular attention should be paid to the radial diameter of the lesion, with a 1-mm to 3-mm margin, in addition to ensuring a full-thickness excision.[4] If malignant melanoma is confirmed by pathologic analysis, reexcision to appropriate margins will likely be required, and consideration of the placement of a marking tattoo or leaving a suture in the skin should be made for small lesions, in the event that reexcision is necessary. Shave biopsies should be avoided, as they frequently do not adequately assess the depth of the lesion. Larger lesions or those in cosmetically sensitive areas, such as the face, should be approached via punch biopsy of the area of darkest pigmentation.[4]

PATHOLOGIC ANALYSIS

Biopsy specimens should be submitted to an expert pathologist for analysis. Melanoma is broadly divided into the following subtypes[6–9]:

- Lentigo maligna melanoma: Arises from the premalignant lentigo maligna lesions, but becomes malignant when they break free of the epidermis and invade the dermis. Frequently diagnosed in the elderly, and are often confused with age spots.
- Superficial spreading melanoma: Most common type of melanoma, characterized by a flat or slightly raised lesion with irregular borders and heterogeneous coloration. Demonstrate radial and vertical growth.
- Acral lentiginous melanoma: Rare and aggressive melanoma that occurs more frequently in African American than white individuals, and is often found on the palms of the hands, soles of feet, or mucus membranes. Due to difficulty in detecting the lesion secondary to location, it frequently presents late.
- Mucosal melanoma: Arises on mucus membranes covered by squamous cells.
- Nodular melanoma: Aggressive tumor that assumes a nodular shape, characterized by an early vertical growth phase with little or no radial growth. Comprises approximately 15% of all malignant melanomas, and are typically smooth and a uniform blue/black color.
- Desmoplastic melanoma: Rare melanoma seen in older adults that is characterized by scant spindle cells and minimal cellular atypia.
- Amelanotic melanoma: Flesh-colored melanoma lesions that lack dark pigmentation.
- Pediatric atypical Spitzoid tumor: Lesion most commonly seen in pediatric or adolescent patients, and characterized by melanocytes that assume a spindled or epithelioid shape.
- Uveal melanoma: Occurs on the uvea or conjunctiva.

Depth of invasion is an important prognostic factor, and is described by Breslow depth as determined by an ocular micrometer to determine maximal tumor thickness and Clark level (**Table 1**).[10,11]

A complete pathologic report by an experienced pathologist is required for accurate histologic analysis of a melanotic lesion. Gross analysis includes a description of the lesion's symmetry, as well as maximum lesion diameter. Complete microscopic assessment should include detailed information regarding the histologic subtype, Clark level, Breslow depth, dermal mitotic rate per square millimeter, degree of atypia,

Table 1 Clark level	
Level	**Anatomic Depth**
Level 1	Melanoma confined to epidermis (in situ)
Level 2	Invasion into the papillary dermis
Level 3	Invasion to the junction of the papillary and reticular dermis
Level 4	Invasion into the reticular dermis
Level 5	Invasion into the subcutaneous fat

From Weedon D. Skin pathology. 2nd edition. Sydney (Australia): Churchill-Livingstone; 2002.

presence of lymphocytic invasion, presence of ulceration or tumor regression, presence of lymphovascular or perineural invasion, microsatellitosis, and margin assessment.[12,13] Tumor thickness/depth of invasion is the most important independent predictor of survival from melanoma, but multiple studies have shown that a high dermal mitotic rate is related to decreased survival, and is second only to tumor thickness in predicting survival.[14–16] The importance in defining mitotic rate accurately is particularly important in thin melanoma, where a single mitosis changes the tumor stage from T1a to T1b.[17] Immunohistochemistry staining for HMB-45, Melan-A protein, anti-phospho-histone 3, and S-100 is frequently performed.[14] If the diagnosis remains in question after routine hematoxylin-eosin (H&E) staining and immunohistochemistry, fluorescent in situ hybridization or comparative genomic hybridization to detect mutational subtypes found in melanocytic tumors can be performed.[18]

ROLE OF SENTINEL LYMPH NODE BIOPSY

The presence of tumor in the lymph nodes is a key prognostic indicator, and accurate identification is paramount for both accurate staging and decision-making on further therapy. If metastases to lymph nodes are identified, lymph node dissection is both prognostic and therapeutic, with improvements in local control and melanoma-specific survival.[19–21]

Initially described by Morton and colleagues,[22] sentinel lymph node biopsy has resolved most of the previous controversies surrounding elective lymph node dissection for clinically node-negative patients. This technique is based on the concept of orderly progression of tumor metastasis through lymphatic channels that are specific to each area of skin that can be followed with appropriate tracers, such as isosulfan blue and Tc-99 labeled sulfur colloid. The sensitivity for detection of tumor in sentinel lymph nodes using blue dye alone is 93%, but approaches 100% when a second tracer (lymphoscintigraphy) is added.[3]

In the setting of clinically nonpalpable nodes, sentinel lymph node biopsy with lymphoscintigraphy is now considered the standard of care in the workup of intermediate-thickness melanoma with a large multicenter randomized study demonstrating its importance in obtaining prognostic information and decreasing regional recurrence.[23] A number of others advocate its use for melanomas with a thickness of 0.76 mm or more, balancing the relative risks of sentinel node biopsy with the information gained.[13,24–26] In addition to lymph node status, the use of sentinel node mapping allows for ultrastaging of the lymph nodes with serial sectioning and immunohistochemistry, which could be impractical with elective lymph node dissections that yield substantially higher numbers of nodes excised. The burden of tumor in the sentinel lymph node is related to melanoma survival, and can be used to determine which patients require completion lymph node dissection. Patients in whom submicrometastases (<0.1 mm) are found in the sentinel node have the same recurrence and survival as sentinel lymph node–negative patients, and can be spared completion lymph node dissection.[27] Patients with micrometastatic deposits (0.1–0.2 mm) in the sentinel node require completion lymph node dissection, because 10% of patients will have additional positive nodes, portending a poorer prognosis and increased risk of death.[27,28] More recently, the utility of completion lymphadenectomy has been questioned as well. A study from the National Cancer Database found that as many as 50% of patients with positive sentinel node dissections do not undergo definitive lymph node dissection.[29] The Multicenter Selective Lymphadenectomy Trial II (MSLT-II), which randomizes patients to completion dissection or observation for positive nodes, has recently finished accruing and will help to answer this question.[30]

SENTINEL LYMPH NODE PROCEDURE

- Preoperative lymphoscintigraphy (particularly for truncal lesions) to localize which nodal basin(s) is/are draining the primary tumor
- Induction of general anesthesia
- Patient positioning and padding of pressure points, with lesion and draining lymph node basins accessible
- Subdermal injection of blue dye around lesion
- Incision over first draining lymph node basin as determined by radioactivity counts
- Identify and isolate blue channel and blue/radioactive lymph node
- Clip lymphatic channels to avoid lymphatic leak
- Remove sentinel lymph nodes, send to pathology

Unlike sentinel lymph node biopsy for breast cancer, sentinel lymph nodes should not typically be sent for frozen section pathologic analysis, but rather sent in their entirety for permanent pathologic examination, as the false-negative rate of frozen analysis of sentinel lymph nodes in melanoma is high.[14] Pathologic evaluation includes standard H&E and immunohistochemistry with staining for HMB-45 and S100[31] and fluorescence in situ hybridization is helpful in distinguishing whether melanocytes in lymph nodes are metastatic melanoma or benign nodal nevi.[32]

IMAGING WORKUP
Chest X-Ray

Routine chest x-ray is frequently used in the initial staging of patients diagnosed with melanoma. However, a number of studies have questioned the cost-effectiveness of this approach. A 2011 study of patients scheduled to undergo sentinel lymph node biopsy for melanoma showed the preoperative chest x-ray did not identify lung metastases, did not change the planned treatment, and did not add any valuable information to the staging workup in any of the 248 patients studied.[33] In the asymptomatic patient, the specificity and sensitivity of routine chest x-ray is low, with a true-positive rate of 0% to 0.5% and false-positive rate of 8% to 15% in large series.[3,34] Furthermore, the performance of routine chest x-rays for patients with asymptomatic, localized melanoma in the United States exceeds $5 million.[3]

Ultrasound

Although the use of ultrasound has been widely used in the preoperative evaluation of lymph nodes in patients with breast cancer, the value of this modality in the assessment of lymph nodes in melanoma is debatable. A small study by De Giorgi and colleagues[35] evaluated the use of contrast-enhanced ultrasound in patients with early-stage melanoma, and reported a negative predictive value of 100%, with all ultrasonographically negative lymph nodes corresponding to sentinel lymph nodes without metastatic disease. However, the study was small, with only 15 patients evaluated. A larger prospective study of 107 patients with melanoma and clinically negative nodes used ultrasound with fine-needle aspiration cytology in the initial assessment of patients with melanoma. The investigators reported a sensitivity of 34% and specificity of 87% in detecting lymph node involvement by ultrasound alone. When fine-needle aspiration and cytology were added to ultrasonographic evaluation, the sensitivity and specificity were 4.7% and 100%, respectively. The investigators concluded that the yield of this diagnostic technique is insufficient for routine use in the evaluation of patients eligible for sentinel lymph node biopsy for melanoma.[36] A study by Marone and colleagues[37] used high-resolution ultrasound before sentinel lymph node biopsy in 623 patients, and showed a positive predictive value of 100% and negative predictive value of 87%. However, the sensitivity of detecting micrometastases was extremely small, and the risk of missing these small melanoma deposits in lymph nodes precludes the use of high-resolution ultrasound as a substitute for sentinel lymph node biopsy.

18-Fluoro-Deoxyglucose Positron Emission Tomography/Computed Tomography

Like other imaging modalities, the use of 18-Fluoro-deoxyglucose positron emission tomography/computed tomography (FDG-PET/CT) has a narrowly defined role in the workup of patients with melanoma. The yield of routine, preoperative radiographic staging (including chest x-ray, bone and liver scans, head CT, upper gastrointestinal series with small-bowel follow-through, or capsule endoscopy) in asymptomatic patients with early-stage melanoma is low.[38,39] Even in asymptomatic patients with stage III melanoma, the *routine* use of staging CT (CT chest/abdomen/pelvis and magnetic resonance imaging [MRI] of the brain) is questionable, with 11 false-positives for every 1 true unsuspected metastasis that is detected.[38] Radiographic workup for occult metastases is indicated in patients presenting with advanced melanoma (late stage III and stage IV), symptomatic patients, or those with persistently elevated lactate dehydrogenase (LDH) levels after initial excision, which suggests the presence of metastatic disease.[40,41] For patients with stage III and IV melanoma, the addition of FDG-PET and whole-body CT to the diagnostic workup was predictive of melanoma-specific survival and disease-free survival.[42] In the setting of palpable lymph nodes, PET/CT was useful in identifying patients whose lymph node disease burden was sufficiently limited as to allow for surgery for local control.[42] In 12% of patients with what was thought to be surgically treatable metastatic melanoma, PET/CT identified metastases missed in conventional imaging, such as CT chest/abdomen/pelvis or brain MRI, ultimately altering the surgical plan.[42] Although PET/CT is not a substitute for sentinel lymph node biopsy in patients with nonpalpable nodes, it does detect macrometastases, and is a useful surgical planning tool.[43] Another study showed that in patients with stage III melanoma, unsuspected metastases were identified by PET/CT in 15% of patients, with a sensitivity of 92% and specificity of 90%.[44] A total of one-third of patients evaluated were upstaged, and two-thirds were downstaged by FDG-PET/CT.[44] Furthermore, a positive PET/CT was the most important predictor of melanoma-specific survival (hazard ratio 2.52) in multivariate analysis, when controlling for gender, lymph node positivity, and extranodal extension. Patients with negative PET/CT scans had 47.6% 5-year melanoma-specific survival, compared with 16.9% for PET/CT-positive patients.[42]

LABORATORY TESTS

Several laboratory tests have been shown to provide prognostic information in selected patients with melanoma. LDH has long been known to be an important predictor of melanoma prognosis. However, a recent study by Wevers and colleagues[45] identified *preoperative* levels of S100-B to be a stronger prognostic biomarker than LDH in patients undergoing lymph node dissection for bulky macrometastatic involvement. Persistent elevated *postoperative* values of LDH remain useful in determining the need for metastatic workup.[40]

For patients with metastatic melanoma, treatment options are few. Recent advances in targeted therapies have identified the BRAF mutation as a potential target, and BRAF inhibitors (ipilimumab) are a therapeutic option in these difficult patients. For patients with stage IV melanoma, evaluation for a BRAF mutation should be performed on the tumor to determine if BRAF inhibitors could be used.[14,46] Surgical excision for oligometastatic disease has also been advocated by some for those with slower doubling times.[47]

Table 2
American Joint Committee on Cancer, seventh edition, staging criteria for cutaneous melanoma

Stage	Description	5-y Survival
Stage 0	In situ	99.9%
Stage I (A/B) T1a: ≤1.0 mm thick, no ulceration, mitosis <1/mm^2 T1b: ≤1.0 mm thick, with ulceration or mitoses ≥1/mm^2 T2a: 1.01–2.0 mm thick, no ulceration	Invasive	89%–95%
Stage II (A, B, C) T2b: 1.01–2.0 mm thick, with ulceration T3a: 2.01–4.0 mm thick, without ulceration T3b: 2.01–4.0 mm thick, with ulceration T4a: >4.0 mm thick, without ulceration T4b: >4.0 mm thick, with ulceration	High risk	45%–79%

Stage III (A, B, C)
N1: Single positive lymph node
  N1a: Micrometastasis
  N1b: Macrometastasis
N2: Two to 3 positive lymph nodes or regional in-transit metastases
  N2a: Micrometastasis
  N2b: Macrometastasis
  N2c: In-transit metastasis/satellites *without* metastatic nodes
N3: Four positive lymph nodes, matted nodes, or in-transit metastases/satellites *with* metastatic nodes
	Regional metastases	24%–70%

Stage IV M1a: Metastases to skin, subcutaneous or distant lymph nodes, normal LDH M1b: Lung metastases, normal LDH M1c: Other visceral metastases or any distant metastases with elevated LDH	Distant metastases	7%–19%

Data from Balch CM, Gershenwald JE, Soong SJ, et al. Melanoma of the skin. In: Edge SB, Byrd DR, Compton CC, editors. AJCC cancer staging manual. 7th edition. New York: Springer; 2010. p. 325–44.

SUMMARY STAGING

Staging of melanoma is based on the 2010 American Joint Committee on Cancer (AJCC) seventh edition TNM system. Unlike previous editions, the most recent AJCC melanoma staging system accounts for the importance of dermal mitotic rate in the prognosis of malignant melanoma. In particular, stage T1b now does not focus solely on ulceration, but includes the presence of one or more mitotic figures per square millimeter and/or ulceration (**Table 2**).[14,48,49]

REFERENCES

1. American Cancer Society. "What are the key statistics about melanoma?". Available at: http://www.cancer.org/cancer/skincancer-melanoma/detailedguide/melanoma-skin-cancer-key-statistics. Accessed March 15, 2014.
2. SEER Stat Fact Sheet: Melanoma. From the National Cancer Institute's Surveillance, Epidemiology, and End Results Database. Available at: http://seer.cancer.gov/statfacts/html/melan.html. Accessed March 15, 2014.
3. Casara D, Rubello D, Rossi CR, et al. Sentinel node biopsy in cutaneous melanoma patients: technical and clinical aspects. Tumori 2000;86(4):339–40.
4. Cameron JL. Current surgical therapy. Philadelphia: Elsevier; 2011.
5. Melanoma. Available at: http://en.wikipedia.org/wiki/Melanoma. Accessed March 15, 2014.
6. James WD, Berger TG, Elston DM. Andrews' diseases of the skin: clinical dermatology. Philadelphia: Saunders Elsevier; 2006.
7. Rapini RP, Bolognia JL, Jorizzo JL. Dermatology: 2-volumme set. St Louis (MO): Mosby; 2007.
8. Leffell DJ. Total skin: the definitive guide to total skin care for life. New Haven (CT): Yale School of Medicine; 2000.
9. Skin- Melanocytic tumor. Available at: http://www.pathologyoutlines.com. Accessed March 24, 2014.
10. Breslow A. Thickness, cross-sectional areas and depth of invasion in the prognosis of cutaneous melanoma. Ann Surg 1970;172(5):902–8.
11. Weedon D. Skin pathology. Sydney (Australia): Churchill-Livingstone; 2002.
12. Reed D, Kudchadkar R, Zager JS, et al. Controversies in the evaluation and management of atypical melanocytic proliferations in children, adolescents, and young adults. J Natl Compr Canc Netw 2013;11(6):679–86.
13. Bichakjian CK, Halpern AC, Johnson TM, et al. Guidelines of care for the management of primary cutaneous melanoma. American Academy of Dermatology. J Am Acad Dermatol 2011;65(5):1032–47.
14. Mathew R, Messina JL. Recent advances in pathologic evaluation and reporting of melanoma. Semin Oncol 2012;39(2):184–91.
15. Sondak VK, Taylor JM, Sabel MS, et al. Mitotic rate and younger age are predictors of sentinel lymph node positivity: lessons learned from a generation of a probabilistic model. Ann Surg Oncol 2004;11(3):247–58.
16. Gouley A. Melanoma staging. Mitotic rate now recognized as the most powerful predictor. Adv NPs PAs 2013;4(5):31–2.
17. Hale CS, Qian M, Ma MW, et al. Mitotic rate in melanoma: prognostic value of immunostaining and computer-assisted image analysis. Am J Surg Pathol 2013; 37(6):882–9.
18. Gerami P, Busam KJ. Cytogenetic and mutational analyses of melanocytic tumors. Dermatol Clin 2012;30(4):555–66.

19. Morton DL, Thompson JF, Cochran AJ, et al. Final trial report of sentinel-node biopsy versus nodal observation in melanoma. N Engl J Med 2014;370(7):599–609.
20. Ross MI, Gershenwald JE. Sentinel lymph node biopsy for melanoma: a critical update for dermatologists after two decades of experience. Clin Dermatol 2013;31(3):298–310.
21. Lotti T, Bruscino N, Hercogova J, et al. Controversial issues on melanoma. Dermatol Ther 2012;25(5):458–62.
22. Morton DL, Wen DR, Wong JH, et al. Technical details of intraoperative lymphatic mapping for early stage melanoma. Arch Surg 1992;127:392–9.
23. Morton DL, Thompson JF, Cochran AJ, et al. Sentinel node biopsy or nodal observation in melanoma. N Engl J Med 2006;355:1307–17.
24. Johnson TM, Bradford CR, Gruber SB, et al. Staging workup, sentinel node biopsy, and follow-up tests for melanoma: update of current concepts. Arch Dermatol 2004;140(1):107–13.
25. Dzwierzynski WW. Managing malignant melanoma. Plast Reconstr Surg 2013; 132(3):446e–60e.
26. Han D, Yu D, Zhao X, et al. Sentinel node biopsy is indicated for thin melanomas > 0.76 mm. Ann Surg Oncol 2012;19(11):3335–42.
27. van Akkooi AC, Nowecki ZI, Voit C, et al. Sentinel node tumor burden according to the Rotterdam criteria is the most important prognostic factor for survival in melanoma patients: a multicenter study in 388 patients with positive sentinel nodes. Ann Surg 2008;248(6):949–55.
28. Leung AM, Morton DL, Ozao-Choy J, et al. Staging of regional lymph nodes in melanoma: a case for including non-sentinel lymph node positivity in the American Joint Committee on Cancer staging system. JAMA Surg 2013;148(9):879–84.
29. Bilimoria KY, Balch CM, Bentrem DJ, et al. Complete lymph node dissection for sentinel node positive melanoma. Ann Surg Oncol 2010;15(6):1566–76.
30. Multicenter selective lymphadenectomy trial II (MSLT-II). Available at: http://clinicaltrials.gov/show/NCT00297895. Accessed March 31, 2014.
31. Blaheta HJ, Sotlar K, Breuninger H, et al. Does intensive histopathological workup by serial sectioning increase the detection of lymph node micrometastasis in patients with primary cutaneous melanoma? Melanoma Res 2001;11(1):57–63.
32. Dalton SR, Gerami P, Kolaitis NA, et al. Use of fluorescence in situ hybridization (FISH) to distinguish intranodal nevus from metastatic melanoma. Am J Surg Pathol 2010;34(2):231–7.
33. Vermeeren L, van der Ent FW, Hulsewe KW. Is there an indication for routine chest x-ray in initial staging of melanoma? J Surg Res 2011;166(1):114–9.
34. Terhune MH, Swanson N, Johnson TM. Use of chest radiography in the initial evaluation of patients with localized melanoma. Arch Dermatol 1998;134(5): 569–72.
35. De Giorgi V, Gori A, Grazzini M, et al. Contrast-enhanced ultrasound: a filter role in AJCC stage I/II melanoma patients. Oncology 2010;79(5–6):370–5.
36. van Rijk MC, Teertstra HJ, Peterse JL, et al. Ultrasonography and fine-needle aspiration cytology in the preoperative evaluation of melanoma patients eligible for sentinel node biopsy. Ann Surg Oncol 2006;13(11):1511–6.
37. Marone U, Catalano O, Caraco C, et al. Can high-resolution ultrasound avoid the sentinel lymph-node biopsy procedure in the staging process of patients with stage I-II cutaneous melanoma? Ultraschall Med 2012;33(7):E179–85.
38. Pandalai PK, Dominguez FJ, Michaelson J, et al. Clinical value of radiographic staging in patients diagnosed with AJCC stage III melanoma. Ann Surg Oncol 2011;18(2):506–13.

39. Prakoso E, Selby WS. Capsule endoscopy in patients with malignant melanoma. Am J Gastroenterol 2007;102(6):1204–8.

40. Khansur T, Sanders J, Das SK. Evaluation of staging workup in malignant melanoma. Arch Surg 1989;124(7):847–9.

41. Orfaniotis G, Mennie JC, Fairbairn N, et al. Findings of computed tomography in stage IIB and IIC melanoma: a six-year retrospective study in the south-east of Scotland. J Plast Reconstr Aesthet Surg 2012;65(9):1216–9.

42. Niebling MG, Bastiaannet E, Hoekstra OS, et al. Outcome of clinical stage III melanoma patients with FDG-PET and whole-body CT added to the diagnostic workup. Ann Surg Oncol 2013;20(9):3098–105.

43. Bourgeois AC, Chang TT, Fish LM, et al. Positron emission tomography/computed tomography in melanoma. Radiol Clin North Am 2013;51(5):865–79.

44. Francis IR, Brown RK, Avram AM. The clinical role of CT/PET in oncology: an update. Cancer Imaging 2005;5:S68–75.

45. Wevers KP, Kruijff S, Speijers MJ, et al. S-100B is a stronger prognostic biomarker than LDH in stage IIIB-C melanoma. Ann Surg Oncol 2013;20(8):2772–9.

46. Moreau S, Saiag P, Aegerter P, et al. Prognostic value of BRAF-V600 mutations in melanoma patients after resection of metastatic lymph nodes. Ann Surg Oncol 2012;19(13):4314–21.

47. Ollila DW, Essner R, Wanek LA, et al. Surgical resection for melanoma metastatic to the gastrointestinal tract. Arch Surg 1996;131:975–80.

48. Piris A, Lobo AC, Duncan LM. Melanoma staging: where are we now? Dermatol Clin 2012;30(4):581–92.

49. Edge S, Byrd DR, Compton CC, et al. AJCC cancer staging manual. 7th edition. Chicago: Springer; 2010.

Principles of Surgical Treatment of Malignant Melanoma

Charles W. Kimbrough, MD, Kelly M. McMasters, MD, PhD,
Eric G. Davis, MD*

KEYWORDS

- Melanoma • Sentinel lymph node biopsy • Completion lymphadenectomy
- Wide local excision

KEY POINTS

- Surgery remains the best chance for cure and regional disease control in patients with melanoma, and most patients will be cured of their disease.
- Multiple randomized controlled trials have established guidelines for adequate resection margins of primary cutaneous melanoma.
- Status of the sentinel lymph node is the most important prognostic factor in patients without clinical nodal disease, and biopsy should be considered in appropriate patients.
- Sentinel lymph node biopsy should be considered for intermediate-thickness (1–4 mm), thick (>4 mm), and high-risk thin melanomas (<1 mm) without clinically involved nodes.
- Completion lymphadenectomy is recommended for patients with tumor-positive sentinel lymph nodes.

INTRODUCTION

Although melanoma represents less than 5% of all skin cancers, it is responsible for the bulk of skin cancer–related deaths.[1] Nevertheless, despite this aggressive reputation, most patients with cutaneous melanoma will be surgically cured of their disease. Early detection allows for curative resection, and 5-year survival for all stages of melanoma is 91%.[2] In patients with early invasive melanoma, 5-year survival rates increase to 97%.[3] Even for those with more advanced disease, the lack of highly effective adjuvant therapy means that surgery still offers the best chance at improved survival or cure. Furthermore, with the incidence increasing at approximately 3% per year, a sound knowledge of the surgical management of melanoma is critical for any general surgeon.[4] This review outlines the surgical treatment of melanoma, including principles of wide local excision (WLE) and management of the regional lymph nodes (**Box 1**).

The Hiram C. Polk, Jr. Department of Surgery, University of Louisville School of Medicine, 550 South Jackson Street, Louisville, KY 40202, USA
* Corresponding author.
E-mail address: egdavi01@louisville.edu

Surg Clin N Am 94 (2014) 973–988
http://dx.doi.org/10.1016/j.suc.2014.07.002
0039-6109/14/$ – see front matter © 2014 Elsevier Inc. All rights reserved.

Box 1
Pearls and pitfalls

Pearls

- SLNB indicated even for thin melanomas in the setting of ulceration or mitotic index greater than $1/mm^2$
- No evidence to suggest margins greater than 2 cm improve recurrence or survival even for thick melanomas
- Fine-needle aspiration is initial step for palpable nodal disease

Pitfalls

- Failure to perform lymphoscintigraphy at the time of SLNB resulting in missed in-transit lymph nodes (epitrochlear, popliteal, and so on)
- Failure to perform therapeutic lymphadenectomy in the setting of palpable metastatic disease with unknown primary melanoma

---

MANAGEMENT OF PRIMARY CUTANEOUS MELANOMA
Background

The aggressive nature of melanoma has long been recognized. Hunter published the first account in 1787, with a case including nodal metastasis. He was followed by Laennec, who noted several visceral metastases and dubbed the disease process "*melanosis*."[5] William Norris reported the "first genuine good case of melanoma" in 1820.[5] Norris[6] may have been the first to endorse WLE and recommended surgery "not only to remove the disease, but to cut away some of the healthy parts." Based on lymphatic spread in a single patient, Handley recommended 5-cm excision margins in 1907.[7] Wide excision with up to 5-cm margins remained the standard of care for more than 50 years, until this dogma came under scrutiny in the 1970s.[8,9] Since then, multiple randomized controlled trials have helped establish contemporary guidelines (**Table 1**).

Thin Melanoma (<1 mm)

One of the earliest challenges to wide excision came in 1977, when Breslow and Macht[10] reported no adverse events in a small series of patients with thin cutaneous melanoma who underwent excision with a narrow margin. Multiple subsequent

---

Table 1
Recommended margins of WLE

Thickness (mm)	WLE Margin (cm)
In situ	0.5–1
<1	1
1–2	1–2[a]
>2–4	2
>4	2[b]

[a] A higher risk of local recurrence may be seen with 1-cm margins in this category.
[b] Larger margins can be considered if there is a high risk of local recurrence, although there is no evidence to suggest greater than 2 cm margins are beneficial.

studies confirmed these findings, and although no randomized controlled trials have addressed excision margins for thin melanomas, the general consensus is that 1-cm margins are sufficient.[11] Looking at pooled data across 5 randomized trials, Lens and colleagues[12] concluded that excision margins of at least 1 cm for thin melanoma did not decrease survival or lead to an increased risk for local recurrence.

Intermediate-Thickness Melanoma (1–4 mm)

Most randomized controlled trials have focused on excision margins for intermediate-thickness melanoma (**Table 2**).[13–18] None have demonstrated a difference in overall survival, disease-free survival (DFS), or local recurrence. Of note, the British Collaborative Trial did find significantly greater locoregional recurrence (pooled local, in-transit, and nodal recurrence) in patients with melanomas greater than 2 mm thick who underwent a 1-cm versus a 3-cm margin.[17] Based on this, a 1-cm margin for melanoma with Breslow thickness greater than 2 mm is considered inadequate. However, margins of 2 cm do appear to be acceptable for these lesions.[18] The World Health Organization (WHO) also reported a nonsignificant increase in local recurrence for melanomas 1 to 2 mm thick that were resected with either 1-cm or 3-cm margins (4.2% vs 1.5%, respectively).[13] Given this trend, 1-cm margins are acceptable but may increase the risk of local recurrence for lesions 1 to 2 mm thick. Excision with 2-cm margins in these patients is adequate, as shown by the Intergroup Melanoma Trial.[16] Driven by these studies, guidelines recommend 2-cm margins for melanoma greater than 2 mm thick, and 1- to 2-cm margins for melanomas 1 to 2 mm thick (see **Table 1**).

Table 2
Randomized-controlled trials assessing resection margins

Trial (Author, Year)	Subjects	Resection Margins (cm) Narrow	Wide	Tumor Thickness (mm)	Site	Findings
WHO (Cascinelli et al,[26] 1998)	612	1	3	0.8–2.0	T, E	No difference in OS, DFS, or LR. 4 local recurrences, all with 1-cm resection margins in melanoma 1–2 mm thick
Swedish (Cohn-Cedermark et al,[14] 2000)	989	2	5	<2	T, E	No difference in OS, DFS, or LR
French (Khayat et al,[15] 2003)	326	2	5	<2.1	T, E, H&N	No difference in OS, DFS, or LR
Intergroup (Balch et al,[39] 2001)	468	2	4	1.0–4.0	T, E	No difference in OS, DFS, or LR
British (Thomas et al,[17] 2004)	900	1	3	>2.0	T, E	No difference in OS, DFS. Increased locoregional (local, in-transit, and nodal) recurrence with 1-cm margins
Swedish/Danish (Gillgren et al,[18] 2011)	936	2	4	>2.0	T, E	No difference in OS, DFS, or LR

Abbreviations: E, extremities; H&N, head and neck; LR, local recurrence; OS, overall survival; T, trunk.

Thick Melanoma (>4 mm)

Limited trial data exist for melanomas greater than 4 mm thick. Based on several retrospective studies, a 2-cm margin appears adequate.[19,20] In a review of 278 patients with tumors greater than 4 mm thick, Heaton and colleagues[19] reported that a 2-cm excision margin had no impact on overall survival, DFS, or local recurrence. Nevertheless, wider excision may be appropriate for thicker lesions with a high risk of local recurrence.[21]

Melanoma in Situ

Melanoma in situ is generally treated with 0.5-cm margins, based largely on clinical experience and a 1992 National Institutes of Health expert consensus statement.[22] However, the adequacy of 0.5 cm as a margin for in situ disease has since been questioned by several studies that demonstrate incomplete resection with this margin size.[23] Initial pathologic evaluation of biopsy specimens can be wrong, with one study demonstrating that expert review of outside pathology specimens led to a change in surgical margins in 12% of early melanomas.[24] For these reasons, it is prudent to perform a 1-cm WLE in anatomic areas that will easily allow primary closure, such as the trunk or extremities.

WLE: Technical Points

- WLE may be performed under local anesthesia, although general anesthesia is generally preferred for patients with planned sentinel lymph node (SLN) biopsy or lymphadenectomy.
- Excision margins are measured from the edge of the lesion or prior biopsy scar and marked. A fusiform incision is usually necessary to allow for primary closure (**Fig. 1**).
- Complete removal of skin and subcutaneous tissue down to the muscular fascia is performed (**Fig. 2**). Excision of the fascia is generally not necessary, but may be considered in patients with thick primary melanomas (>4 mm).
- Undermining of the skin can be performed to allow for primary closure without unnecessary tension. Skin grafts and complex adjacent tissue rearrangement are not usually necessary, but may be required for lesions of the head and neck or distal extremities.
- The specimen is submitted for permanent section; no frozen section analysis of margins should be attempted. Adequate margins are determined clinically at the time of excision, and re-excision is not necessary if final pathology indicates the measured margin is less than the recommended margin. Involved or nearly involved margins on final pathology warrant re-excision.

MANAGEMENT OF THE REGIONAL LYMPH NODES
Background

Analogous to resection of the primary lesion, management of the regional lymph nodes has been refined over the years from initial aggressive strategies. In 1892, Herbert Snow reported a predilection for cutaneous melanoma to spread to the regional lymph nodes. Snow recognized that melanoma spread first to the regional lymph nodes, and that bulky nodal disease increased the risk of distant disease.[5] As such, he recommended elective lymphadenectomy in the treatment of melanoma, a topic that remained controversial for more than a century.

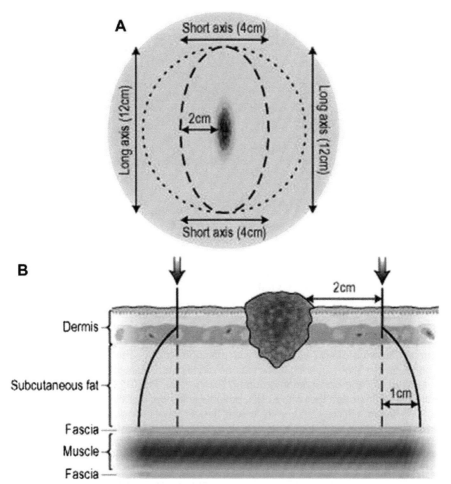

Fig. 1. (*A*) With 2-cm margins, a 3:1 ratio of length to width yields a long axis of 12 cm, resulting in dimensions for an adequate fusiform excision. (*B*) The creation of flaps by raising a plane that extends at least 1 cm above the deep muscle fascia helps with a tension-free closure. (*From* Andtbacka RH. Surgical excision of melanoma. In: Rigel DS, Robinson JK, Ross MI, et al, editors. Cancer of the skin. 2nd edition. Philadelphia: Elsevier; 2011: 532–5; with permission.)

Elective Lymphadenectomy

Snow's initial observations were prescient in that patients will rarely present with distant disease without first developing nodal metastasis. Approximately 20% of patients with primary lesions greater than 1 mm thick will go on to develop palpable nodal disease if left untreated. Proponents of elective lymph node dissection (ELND) argued early resection held a survival advantage for this subset of patients. However, given that 80% of patients will not develop nodal disease, opponents to ELND argued that most patients were unnecessarily exposed to the significant morbidity of lymphadenectomy. Instead, they supported therapeutic lymph node dissection (TLND), performed once nodal disease became clinically apparent.

The controversy between elective and TLND ultimately led to several randomized controlled trials. Although none demonstrated an overall survival benefit for ELND, 2

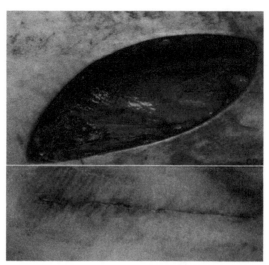

Fig. 2. Fusiform WLE down to muscle fascia (*top*). Raising flaps allows for tension-free closure (*bottom*). (*From* McMasters KM, Urist MM. Melanoma and cutaneous malignancies. In: Townsend CM, Beauchamp RD, Evers BM, et al, editors. Sabiston textbook of surgery. 19th edition. Philadelphia: Elsevier; 2012. p. 742–67; with permission.)

studies warrant discussion for their findings on subgroup analysis. The Intergroup Melanoma Trial randomized 740 patients with melanomas 1 to 4 mm thick to either ELND or nodal observation. Overall, there was no significant difference in 10-year survival between ELND and observation groups (77% vs 72%, *P* = .12). However, subgroup analysis demonstrated that with ELND, patients with nonulcerated melanomas, melanomas 1 to 2 mm thick, or extremity lesions had a reduction in mortality of 30%, 30%, and 27%, respectively.[25] In the second study, no survival benefit was seen in a WHO trial comparing ELND with nodal observation in 240 patients with truncal melanomas greater than 1.5 mm thick. However, patients with occult nodal disease detected by ELND had a significant improvement in 5-year survival over patients who developed nodal disease under observation and required TLND (48% vs 27%, *P* = .04). This subgroup analysis suggested that early resection of microscopic nodal metastasis may improve survival.[26]

SLN Biopsy

In 1977, the late Dr Donald Morton described a new technique to identify the principal nodal basin receiving lymphatic drainage from truncal melanomas.[27] These lesions potentially drain to several different nodal basins, and before SLN biopsy, the decision of which nodal basin to dissect electively was based on Sappey lines, which were derived from anatomic studies in the 19th century. With lymphoscintigraphy, radioactive tracer injected into the dermis surrounding a melanoma is absorbed by the adjacent lymphatic channels and subsequently can be localized within the first draining lymph nodes.

From the initial report in 1977, nodal mapping was refined to allow intraoperative identification of the sentinel node. The concept of the sentinel node was based on the theory that the first draining nodes would also be the first to receive metastatic spread from the primary tumor (**Fig. 3**). In the early 1990s, Morton and colleagues[28] were able to show that the sentinel node accurately determined the status of the entire

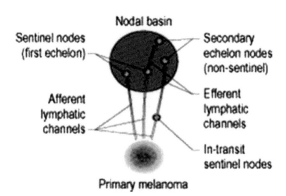

Fig. 3. Afferent lymphatic channels initially drain to first echelon nodes (sentinel nodes) before proceeding to secondary (nonsentinel) nodes. Interval (in-transit) nodes may occur between the primary melanoma and the nodal basin. (*From* Ross MI. Regional lymph node surgery in melanoma patients. In: Rigel DS, Robinson JK, Ross MI, et al, editors. Cancer of the skin. 2nd edition. Philadelphia: Elsevier; 2011. p. 544–58; with permission.)

draining nodal basin with a low false-negative rate. The study proved the theory of the sentinel node: nonsentinel nodes were the only site of metastasis in 2 of 3079 nodes collected from 187 lymph node dissection (LND) specimens.[28] SLN biopsy was further validated by numerous studies that followed.

Clinical Evidence for SLN Biopsy

In a landmark paper, Gershenwald and colleagues[29] demonstrated that the sentinel node is the most important prognostic factor in patients without clinical evidence of nodal disease. Successful identification of the sentinel node has become critical for prognosis and staging. By identifying patients with occult nodal metastases, SLN biopsy may help prevent progression of regional nodal disease and identify patients who need additional therapy, such as completion lymphadenectomy.[30]

Many articles have assessed SLN biopsy, and a comprehensive meta-analysis combined 71 of these studies involving 25,240 patients to evaluate its validity and reliability as a procedure. Overall, the rate of successful SLN identification was 98.1%, with a false negative rate of 12.5%.[31] The estimated risk for nodal recurrence after a negative SLN biopsy was less than 5%. Furthermore, as a minimally invasive procedure, studies indicate SLN biopsy results in fewer complications than lymphadenectomy. The Sunbelt Melanoma Trial and the first Multicenter Selective Lymphadenectomy Trial (MSLT I) estimated complication rates from SLN biopsy as 4.6% and 10.1%, respectively.[32,33] As such, SLN biopsy offers the same prognostic information as ELND with much less morbidity.

The only randomized control trial to evaluate outcomes of SLN biopsy versus nodal observation is MSLT I, initiated by Morton in 1994. A total of 1347 patients with intermediate-thickness melanoma (1.2–3.5 mm thick) were randomized to either SLN biopsy or observation. An additional 314 patients with thick melanoma (>3.5 mm thick) were also randomized. In the final trial report, no difference was seen in 10-year melanoma-specific survival between SLN biopsy and observation in either the intermediate thickness (81.4% vs 78.3%, $P = .18$) or the thick melanoma groups (58.9% vs 64.4%, $P = .56$).[34] However, improved 10-year DFS was seen in both groups. Among patients with intermediate-thickness melanoma, DFS was 71.3% with SLN biopsy, compared with 64.7% for observation ($P = .01$). For thick melanoma, the respective DFS rates were 50.7% and 40.5% ($P = .03$). In patients that underwent SLN biopsy, sentinel node status was the strongest predictor of recurrence or death from melanoma. With a negative sentinel node, 10-year survival was 85.1%, compared with 62.1% for those with positive biopsies (hazard ratio [HR] 3.09, 95% CI 2.12–4.49, P<.001).[34]

Indications

As with any procedure, the decision to perform SLN biopsy requires balancing the risk versus potential benefit. Although SLN biopsy is a minimally invasive procedure, there are associated costs and complication rates. Given the results from MSLT-1, and the fact that approximately 20% of patients with intermediate-thickness melanoma will have metastasis to regional nodes, it is well established that SLN biopsy is appropriate for these patients.[35] However, there has been some controversy regarding the role of SLN biopsy in patients with either thick or thin melanoma (**Table 3**).

Thick melanomas

Because patients with thick melanoma are at increased risk for distant metastatic disease, prior dogma has suggested that these patients would not benefit from SLN biopsy or LND. However, if no distant disease is present, these patients should be managed similarly to those with intermediate-thickness melanomas.[35] In one review of 240 patients with melanomas greater than 4 mm thick, 58% of patients had a negative SLN biopsy, and those with a negative biopsy had both improved distant DFS and overall survival compared with patients with a positive node.[36] Given that disease progression is a continuum, and that lesions greater than 4 mm do not necessarily indicate distant spread, SLN biopsy in thick melanoma could provide improved regional disease control and possibly cure in some patients.

Thin melanomas

Up to 70% of melanomas in the United States present as thin melanoma.[37] Overall, the risk of nodal metastasis in these patients is estimated at only 5% or less, and routine use of SLN biopsy is not indicated.[38] However, subsets of this population can have rates of sentinel node positivity that approach those seen with intermediate-thickness lesions. The precise identification of high-risk populations and defining the role for SLN biopsy in these patients have been controversial topics and continue to evolve.

Several features of the primary lesion have been linked to an increased risk of nodal metastasis. In particular, ulceration and mitotic rate (≥ 1 mitosis/mm^2) have been identified as strong predictors of nodal disease in patients with thin melanomas. In fact, a review of 4861 T1 melanomas from the American Joint Committee of Cancer (AJCC) database found that mitotic rate was the most powerful predictor of survival in these

Table 3 Recommendations for SLN biopsy	
Thickness	**Recommendation**
Intermediate (1–4 mm)	Perform SLN biopsy
Thick (>4 mm)	Perform SLN biopsy
Thin (<1 mm)	Routine biopsy not indicated. Consider in high-risk patients with ulceration, mitotic rate ≥ 1/mm^2, or select lesions >0.75 mm thick

Adapted from Wong SL, Balch CM, Hurley P, et al. Sentinel lymph node biopsy for melanoma: American Society of Clinical Oncology and Society of Surgical Oncology joint clinical practice guideline. J Clin Oncol 2012;30(23):2912–8.

patients.[39] In addition, multiple studies have indicated ulceration as a risk factor for SLN metastasis.[40–42] As such, both ulceration and mitotic rate were incorporated into the seventh edition of the AJCC staging system to discriminate T1a from T1b lesions.[2] Considered stage IB lesions, it is recommended that patients with T1b melanomas be considered for SLN biopsy.[38,43]

Additional consideration for biopsy can be based on the thickness of the primary lesion. Lesions less than 0.75 mm thick have a SLN metastasis rate of 2.7%, compared with 6.2% for lesions greater than 0.75 mm. Therefore, routine SLN biopsy of lesions less than 0.75 mm cannot be recommended in the absence of additional factors associated with a poor prognosis.[38] Although some suggest SLN biopsy is indicated for all lesions greater than 0.75 mm, there is no general consensus.[42] Patients with high-risk features such as ulceration or mitotic rate greater than or equal to $1/mm^2$ with melanomas greater than 0.75 mm should have strong consideration for SLN biopsy. Although Clark level alone may not be sufficiently predictive to warrant SLN biopsy, biopsy should be considered for Clark level IV/V invasion present in combination with other high-risk features, such as ulceration, mitotic rate, or Breslow depth.[38,39] Younger patients are at increased risk for SLN metastasis in some models, but no clear age cutoff has been established.[44] SLN biopsy may be reasonable in patients younger than 40 if other high-risk factors are present.[38] Similarly, male gender can indicate increased risk in the presence of other high-risk factors. For instance, men with thin melanomas greater than 0.75 mm thick and a mitotic rate greater than zero have an estimated SLN metastasis rate of 16.1%.[45]

SLN Biopsy Technical Points

Lymphoscintigraphy

- All patients should undergo preoperative lymphoscintigraphy on the same day as WLE and SLN biopsy. Radioactive tracer (Technetium-99 sulfur colloid) is injected into the dermis surrounding the melanoma or biopsy site, raising a small wheal. Injections should be performed 0.5 cm away from the primary lesion or biopsy site to avoid any lymphatics disrupted by the tumor or biopsy procedure.
- Injecting too deeply into the subcutaneous tissue may lead to false-negative imaging. If the initial injection does not identify any sentinel nodes, repeat injection should be performed by an experienced practitioner.
- Imaging will occasionally identify sentinel nodes in more than one nodal basin or identify nodes outside of the traditional cervical, axillary, or inguinal nodal regions. This region includes so-called interval or in-transit nodes, which can contain metastatic foci of disease at nearly the same frequency as traditional nodal basins. Furthermore, in up to 85% of cases where the interval node is positive, it will be the only site of metastatic disease.[46] All identified sentinel nodes, including interval nodes, should be removed (**Fig. 4**).

Sentinel node biopsy

- SLN biopsy is usually performed under general anesthesia. Dermal injection of a vital blue dye (isosulfan blue) is performed with a technique similar to that used for radioactive tracer (**Fig. 5**).
- Depending on the size of the melanoma, injection of 1 to 5 mL of dye is generally sufficient. Injection should be performed within the margins of the planned WLE, as blue dye will persist in the skin for months after injection. Dye does not last nearly as long in sentinel nodes, and therefore, injection should be performed just before incision.

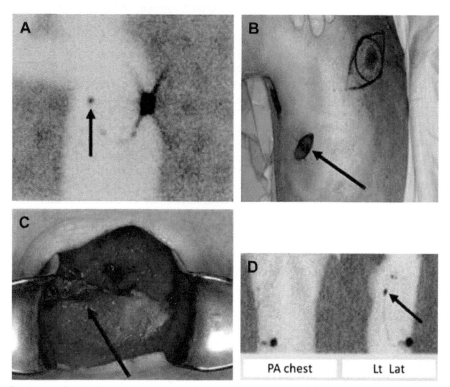

Fig. 4. Lymphoscintigraphy demonstrating an in-transit node (*A*). Operative views demonstrate the node location in relation to the primary and draining nodal basin (*B*) with a blue node and afferent lymphatics evident on close-up view (*C*). A similar lymphoscintigraphy pattern with an in-transit node was seen in another patient (*D*). The *arrow* indicates blue lymphatic channels leading into a blue lymph node. (*From* Ross MI, Gershenwald JE. Sentinel lymph node biopsy for melanoma: a critical update for dermatologists after two decades of experience. Clin Dermatol 2013;31(3):298–310; with permission.)

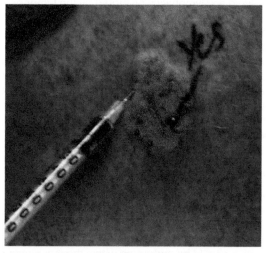

Fig. 5. Intradermal injection of isosulfan blue before SLN biopsy. (*From* McMasters KM, Urist MM. Melanoma and cutaneous malignancies. In: Townsend CM, Beauchamp RD, Evers BM, et al, editors. Sabiston textbook of surgery. 19th edition. Philadelphia: Elsevier; 2012. p. 742–67; with permission.)

- A handheld gamma probe is used to identify the area of the sentinel node, with further dissection guided by any blue lymphatic channels (**Fig. 6**). The most radioactive node, any blue nodes, nodes clinically suspicious for cancer, and nodes with a radioactive count 10% or greater than the most radioactive node are considered sentinel nodes and require resection.[47]
- SLN specimens should be sent for permanent section with immunohistochemical stains for melanoma markers (eg, S-100, HMB-45). Frozen section is to be avoided, because micrometastatic foci are difficult to diagnose on frozen section even by expert pathologists. If the patient will require completion lymphadenectomy, it can be performed at a later operation.

LND Lymph Node Dissection

Completion lymph node dissection

Current guidelines recommend completion lymph node dissection (CLND) for patients with metastasis identified by SLN biopsy, based in part on the increased risk of nodal recurrence if lymphadenectomy is not performed.[35] In a review of patients with a positive SLN biopsy who did not undergo CLND, Wong and colleagues[48] found nodal disease as a site of first recurrence in 15% of patients. From this and other studies, it is reasonable to assume that nodal recurrence after a positive SLN biopsy without CLND

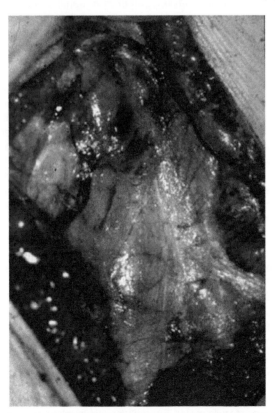

Fig. 6. Lymphatic channels stained blue leading to the sentinel node. (*From* McMasters KM, Urist MM. Melanoma and cutaneous malignancies. In: Townsend CM, Beauchamp RD, Evers BM, et al, editors. Sabiston textbook of surgery. 19th edition. Philadelphia: Elsevier; 2012. p. 742–67; with permission.)

is around 15%.[35] In contrast, data from the Sunbelt Melanoma Trial demonstrated a 4.9% rate of regional nodal recurrence after completion lymphadenectomy, and a similar rate of 4.2% was reported in MSLT I.[49,50]

In addition to improved regional disease control, a second goal of CLND is improved survival. Although currently there is no direct evidence that CLND improves survival, subgroup analysis of MSLT I suggests a benefit for management with SLN biopsy followed by CLND. Ten-year melanoma-specific survival was 62.1% in patients with positive sentinel nodes who immediately underwent CLND, compared with 41.5% in patients under observation who required delayed therapeutic lymphadenectomy (HR 0.56, $P = .006$).[34] Future insight regarding the role of CLND will come from the Multicenter Selective Lymphadenectomy Trial II (MSLT II), which randomizes patients with a tumor-positive SLN to immediate CLND or observation.

Nevertheless, some physicians have challenged the necessity of CLND, and an estimated 50% of patients with a positive sentinel node may not undergo the procedure.[51,52] Opponents argue that there is no clear evidence that CLND improves overall survival, and because approximately 80% of patients ultimately have negative nonsentinel nodes, most patients are unnecessarily exposed to the significant morbidity of a LND.[51] This unnecessary exposure has led to multiple attempts to identify predictors of nonsentinel node metastasis in patients with a positive SLN biopsy.[51,53,54] Although tumor burden within the sentinel node appears to be predictive of nonsentinel node disease, no clear guidelines have been established.[55] Until evidence-based guidelines or results from MSLT II become available, CLND remains the standard of care following a positive SLN biopsy.

TLND

Approximately 4% to 9% of patients presenting with melanoma will have palpable nodal disease, and additional patients may have suspicious nodes on imaging studies.[56] All patients with nodes concerning for metastasis should undergo fine-needle aspiration biopsy, as in some cases these nodes will be benign and do not require resection. Occasionally, patients will also present with involved regional lymph nodes from an unknown primary melanoma. The absence of a primary lesion does not preclude surgery, and therapeutic lymphadenectomy is still indicated in this setting.[56] Interestingly, patients without a primary lesion have better postoperative survival than those with a known lesion, suggesting they may have had a stronger immune response against the primary melanoma.[57]

Technical points

- Lymphadenectomy for melanoma should be as complete as possible, and failure to completely clear nodes is a frequent cause of nodal recurrence in these patients. Goals of surgery include regional disease control and cure, and unlike diseases such as breast cancer, adjuvant therapy cannot be relied on to improve regional disease control.
- Axillary dissection mandates removal of level I, II, and III nodes, including dissection cephalad to the axillary vein. All fibrofatty tissue around the vein, the thoracodorsal and medial pectoral neurovascular bundles, and the long thoracic nerve should be removed. Removal of bulky nodes may require division of the pectoralis minor at the coracoid process and on rare occasions may necessitate division of the pectoralis major. For axillary vein involvement, ligation with resection of involved vein segments may be necessary.
- Inguinal node dissection includes both superficial inguinal and deep (pelvic) nodes, although in most cases, superficial inguinal LND is sufficient for patients with

a tumor-positive SLN. Indications for dissection of pelvic (internal iliac, external iliac, and obturator) nodes vary. Generally, patients who present with palpable superficial inguinal nodal disease require pelvic dissection. Additional indications have included involvement of pelvic nodes on preoperative imaging, multiple positive nodes on superficial dissection, or metastasis to the most cephalad of the deep inguinal lymph nodes, known as Cloquet's node.[58]

SUMMARY

Surgery remains the cornerstone of effective therapy for malignant melanoma, and most patients will be cured of their disease. Through steady accumulation of evidence and randomized controlled trials, radical resection and elective lymphadenectomy have given way to more refined management algorithms. Current guidelines for WLE and the appropriate use of SLN biopsy to guide management of the nodal basin have improved patient outcomes while minimizing morbidity. As more is learned regarding the tumor biology and behavior of melanoma, adherence to evidence-based practice will be critical in providing the best surgical care for these patients.

REFERENCES

1. Miller AJ, Mihm MC Jr. Melanoma. N Engl J Med 2006;355(1):51–65.
2. Balch CM, Gershenwald JE, Soong SJ, et al. Final version of 2009 AJCC melanoma staging and classification. J Clin Oncol 2009;27(36):6199–206.
3. American Cancer Society. Cancer Facts & Figures 2014. Atlanta (GA): American Cancer Society; 2014.
4. Linos E, Swetter SM, Cockburn MG, et al. Increasing burden of melanoma in the United States. J Invest Dermatol 2009;129(7):1666–74.
5. Neuhaus SJ, Clark MA, Thomas JM. Dr. Herbert Lumley Snow, MD, MRCS (1847-1930): the original champion of elective lymph node dissection in melanoma. Ann Surg Oncol 2004;11(9):875–8.
6. Norris W. Eight cases of melanosis with pathological and therapeutic remarks on that disease. London: Longman, Brown, Green, Longman, and Roberts; 1857.
7. Eedy DJ. Surgical treatment of melanoma. Br J Dermatol 2003;149(1):2–12.
8. Wong CK. A study of melanocytes in the normal skin surrounding malignant melanomata. Dermatologica 1970;141(3):215–25.
9. Ross MI, Gershenwald JE. Evidence-based treatment of early-stage melanoma. J Surg Oncol 2011;104(4):341–53.
10. Breslow A, Macht SD. Optimal size of resection margin for thin cutaneous melanoma. Surg Gynecol Obstet 1977;145(5):691–2.
11. Bichakjian CK, Halpern AC, Johnson TM, et al. Guidelines of care for the management of primary cutaneous melanoma. American Academy of Dermatology. J Am Acad Dermatol 2011;65(5):1032–47.
12. Lens MB, Nathan P, Bataille V. Excision margins for primary cutaneous melanoma: updated pooled analysis of randomized controlled trials. Arch Surg 2007;142(9):885–91 [discussion: 891–3].
13. Cascinelli N. Margin of resection in the management of primary melanoma. Semin Surg Oncol 1998;14(4):272–5.
14. Cohn-Cedermark G, Rutqvist LE, Andersson R, et al. Long term results of a randomized study by the Swedish Melanoma Study Group on 2-cm versus 5-cm resection margins for patients with cutaneous melanoma with a tumor thickness of 0.8-2.0 mm. Cancer 2000;89(7):1495–501.

15. Khayat D, Rixe O, Martin G, et al. Surgical margins in cutaneous melanoma (2 cm versus 5 cm for lesions measuring less than 2.1-mm thick). Cancer 2003;97(8):1941–6.
16. Balch CM, Soong SJ, Smith T, et al. Long-term results of a prospective surgical trial comparing 2 cm vs. 4 cm excision margins for 740 patients with 1-4 mm melanomas. Ann Surg Oncol 2001;8(2):101–8.
17. Thomas JM, Newton-Bishop J, A'Hern R, et al. Excision margins in high-risk malignant melanoma. N Engl J Med 2004;350(8):757–66.
18. Gillgren P, Drzewiecki KT, Niin M, et al. 2-cm versus 4-cm surgical excision margins for primary cutaneous melanoma thicker than 2 mm: a randomised, multicentre trial. Lancet 2011;378(9803):1635–42.
19. Heaton KM, Sussman JJ, Gershenwald JE, et al. Surgical margins and prognostic factors in patients with thick (>4 mm) primary melanoma. Ann Surg Oncol 1998;5(4):322–8.
20. Pasquali S, Haydu LE, Scolyer RA, et al. The importance of adequate primary tumor excision margins and sentinel node biopsy in achieving optimal locoregional control for patients with thick primary melanomas. Ann Surg 2013; 258(1):152–7.
21. Mocellin S, Pasquali S, Nitti D. The impact of surgery on survival of patients with cutaneous melanoma: revisiting the role of primary tumor excision margins. Ann Surg 2011;253(2):238–43.
22. Sober AJ. Diagnosis and management of early melanoma: a consensus view. Semin Surg Oncol 1993;9(3):194–7.
23. Kunishige JH, Brodland DG, Zitelli JA. Margins for standard excision of melanoma in situ. J Am Acad Dermatol 2013;69(1):164.
24. Santillan AA, Messina JL, Marzban SS, et al. Pathology review of thin melanoma and melanoma in situ in a multidisciplinary melanoma clinic: impact on treatment decisions. J Clin Oncol 2010;28(3):481–6.
25. Balch CM, Soong S, Ross MI, et al. Long-term results of a multi-institutional randomized trial comparing prognostic factors and surgical results for intermediate thickness melanomas (1.0 to 4.0 mm). Intergroup Melanoma Surgical Trial. Ann Surg Oncol 2000;7(2):87–97.
26. Cascinelli N, Morabito A, Santinami M, et al. Immediate or delayed dissection of regional nodes in patients with melanoma of the trunk: a randomised trial. WHO Melanoma Programme. Lancet 1998;351(9105):793–6.
27. Robinson DS, Sample WF, Fee HJ, et al. Regional lymphatic drainage in primary malignant melanoma of the trunk determined by colloidal gold scanning. Surg Forum 1977;28:147–8.
28. Morton DL, Wen DR, Wong JH, et al. Technical details of intraoperative lymphatic mapping for early stage melanoma. Arch Surg 1992;127(4):392–9.
29. Gershenwald JE, Thompson W, Mansfield PF, et al. Multi-institutional melanoma lymphatic mapping experience: the prognostic value of sentinel lymph node status in 612 stage I or II melanoma patients. J Clin Oncol 1999;17(3):976–83.
30. Gershenwald JE, Ross MI. Sentinel-lymph-node biopsy for cutaneous melanoma. N Engl J Med 2011;364(18):1738–45.
31. Valsecchi ME, Silbermins D, de Rosa N, et al. Lymphatic mapping and sentinel lymph node biopsy in patients with melanoma: a meta-analysis. J Clin Oncol 2011;29(11):1479–87.
32. Morton DL, Cochran AJ, Thompson JF, et al. Sentinel node biopsy for early-stage melanoma: accuracy and morbidity in MSLT-I, an international multicenter trial. Ann Surg 2005;242(3):302–11 [discussion: 311–3].

33. Wrightson WR, Wong SL, Edwards MJ, et al. Complications associated with sentinel lymph node biopsy for melanoma. Ann Surg Oncol 2003;10(6):676–80.
34. Morton DL, Thompson JF, Cochran AJ, et al. Final trial report of sentinel-node biopsy versus nodal observation in melanoma. N Engl J Med 2014;370(7):599–609.
35. Wong SL, Balch CM, Hurley P, et al. Sentinel lymph node biopsy for melanoma: American Society of Clinical Oncology and Society of Surgical Oncology joint clinical practice guideline. J Clin Oncol 2012;30(23):2912–8.
36. Scoggins CR, Bowen AL, Martin RC 2nd, et al. Prognostic information from sentinel lymph node biopsy in patients with thick melanoma. Arch Surg 2010; 145(7):622–7.
37. Criscione VD, Weinstock MA. Melanoma thickness trends in the United States, 1988-2006. J Invest Dermatol 2010;130(3):793–7.
38. Andtbacka RH, Gershenwald JE. Role of sentinel lymph node biopsy in patients with thin melanoma. J Natl Compr Canc Netw 2009;7(3):308–17.
39. Balch CM, Gershenwald JE, Soong SJ, et al. Update on the melanoma staging system: the importance of sentinel node staging and primary tumor mitotic rate. J Surg Oncol 2011;104(4):379–85.
40. Rousseau DL Jr, Ross MI, Johnson MM, et al. Revised American Joint Committee on Cancer staging criteria accurately predict sentinel lymph node positivity in clinically node-negative melanoma patients. Ann Surg Oncol 2003;10(5):569–74.
41. Yonick DV, Ballo RM, Kahn E, et al. Predictors of positive sentinel lymph node in thin melanoma. Am J Surg 2011;201(3):324–7 [discussion: 327–8].
42. Han D, Zager JS, Shyr Y, et al. Clinicopathologic predictors of sentinel lymph node metastasis in thin melanoma. J Clin Oncol 2013;31(35):4387–93.
43. Vaquerano J, Kraybill WG, Driscoll DL, et al. American Joint Committee on Cancer clinical stage as a selection criterion for sentinel lymph node biopsy in thin melanoma. Ann Surg Oncol 2006;13(2):198–204.
44. Sondak VK, Wong SL, Gershenwald JE, et al. Evidence-based clinical practice guidelines on the use of sentinel lymph node biopsy in melanoma. Am Soc Clin Oncol Educ Book 2013;320–5.
45. Kesmodel SB, Karakousis GC, Botbyl JD, et al. Mitotic rate as a predictor of sentinel lymph node positivity in patients with thin melanomas. Ann Surg Oncol 2005;12(6):449–58.
46. McMasters KM, Chao C, Wong SL, et al. Interval sentinel lymph nodes in melanoma. Arch Surg 2002;137(5):543–7 [discussion: 547–9].
47. McMasters KM, Reintgen DS, Ross MI, et al. Sentinel lymph node biopsy for melanoma: how many radioactive nodes should be removed? Ann Surg Oncol 2001;8(3):192–7.
48. Wong SL, Morton DL, Thompson JF, et al. Melanoma patients with positive sentinel nodes who did not undergo completion lymphadenectomy: a multi-institutional study. Ann Surg Oncol 2006;13(6):809–16.
49. Morton DL, Thompson JF, Cochran AJ, et al. Sentinel-node biopsy or nodal observation in melanoma. N Engl J Med 2006;355(13):1307–17.
50. McMasters KM, Noyes RD, Reintgen DS, et al. Lessons learned from the Sunbelt Melanoma Trial. J Surg Oncol 2004;86(4):212–23.
51. van der Ploeg AP, van Akkooi AC, Verhoef C, et al. Completion lymph node dissection after a positive sentinel node: no longer a must? Curr Opin Oncol 2013;25(2):152–9.
52. Bilimoria KY, Balch CM, Bentrem DJ, et al. Complete lymph node dissection for sentinel node-positive melanoma: assessment of practice patterns in the United States. Ann Surg Oncol 2008;15(6):1566–76.

53. Nagaraja V, Eslick GD. Is complete lymph node dissection after a positive sentinel lymph node biopsy for cutaneous melanoma always necessary? A meta-analysis. Eur J Surg Oncol 2013;39(7):669–80.

54. Murali R, Desilva C, Thompson JF, et al. Non-Sentinel Node Risk Score (N-SNORE): a scoring system for accurately stratifying risk of non-sentinel node positivity in patients with cutaneous melanoma with positive sentinel lymph nodes. J Clin Oncol 2010;28(29):4441–9.

55. Cadili A, McKinnon G, Wright F, et al. Validation of a scoring system to predict non-sentinel lymph node metastasis in melanoma. J Surg Oncol 2010;101(3):191–4.

56. Prens SP, van der Ploeg AP, van Akkooi AC, et al. Outcome after therapeutic lymph node dissection in patients with unknown primary melanoma site. Ann Surg Oncol 2011;18(13):3586–92.

57. Lee CC, Faries MB, Wanek LA, et al. Improved survival after lymphadenectomy for nodal metastasis from an unknown primary melanoma. J Clin Oncol 2008; 26(4):535–41.

58. Mack LA, McKinnon JG. Controversies in the management of metastatic melanoma to regional lymphatic basins. J Surg Oncol 2004;86(4):189–99.

Surviving Cutaneous Melanoma

A Clinical Review of Follow-up Practices, Surveillance, and Management of Recurrence

Amy A. Mrazek, MD[a], Celia Chao, MD[b],*

KEYWORDS

- Melanoma survivorship • Survival prognosis • Surveillance and follow-up
- Management of recurrence

KEY POINTS

- Surveillance strategies should be more frequent for patients with advanced stages of melanoma, and visit frequency can decrease over time as the disease-free interval increases.
- Important components of follow-up examinations include history and physical examinations, patient education, risk factor modification, assessment of the psychosocial impact of disease, and counseling on healthy coping mechanisms.
- The work-up of melanoma recurrence is based on the type of recurrence: local, satellite/in-transit, regional, or distant metastatic disease.
- The treatment of melanoma recurrence parallels how primary tumors, nodal, and distant metastases are managed.

INTRODUCTION

In the past 10 years, the incidence of melanoma in the United States has been increasing an average of 2.6% each year, while the death rates have remained stable over time.[1] Furthermore, a similar trend has been observed on a global scale within the last 2 decades, with the highest incidences of melanoma in Australia and New Zealand.[2,3] According to the latest report by the National Cancer Institute's Surveillance, Epidemiology, and End Results (SEER) program, an estimated 921,780 people living in the United States have survived melanoma, and their overall 5- and 10-year relative survival rates are 91.3% and 89.1%, respectively.[1] Most melanoma cases are

Disclosures: All of the authors have no conflicts of interests to disclose.
[a] Department of Surgery, University of Texas Medical Branch, 301 University Boulevard, Route 0534, Galveston, TX 77555, USA; [b] Department of Surgery, University of Texas Medical Branch, 301 University Boulevard, Route 0737, Galveston, TX 77555, USA
* Corresponding author.
E-mail address: cechao@utmb.edu

Surg Clin N Am 94 (2014) 989–1002
http://dx.doi.org/10.1016/j.suc.2014.07.003
0039-6109/14/$ – see front matter © 2014 Elsevier Inc. All rights reserved.

surgical.theclinics.com

diagnosed at a localized stage, which have more favorable survival rates (98.3%) compared with those with regional (62.4%) or distant metastatic disease (16.0%).[1]

A major component of survivorship involves follow-up and monitoring for recurrence and/or new malignancies. Yang and colleagues[4] reviewed the SEER database from 1988 to 2007, focusing on the relative risk (RR) of developing a second primary cutaneous melanoma (CM) in 70,819 melanoma survivors and 6353 patients with CM subsequent to another primary malignancy. No matter the age of initial melanoma diagnosis, survivors had an increased risk of recurrence: RR 11.89, 95% confidence interval (CI), 10.83 to 13.03, for patients younger than 45 years and RR 8.36, 95% CI, 7.93 to 8.81, for patients at least 45 years of age. Furthermore, the RR remained elevated for the duration of the 15-year study period.[4] These results reinforce the importance of surveillance to identify early and treat new primary CM in previous melanoma survivors.[5]

PROGNOSTIC FACTORS FOR MELANOMA SURVIVAL

The American Joint Committee on Cancer (AJCC) Melanoma Task Force has collected data from 30,946 patients, spanning multiple institutions and continents, to develop an evidence-based staging system that helps clinicians evaluate patient prognosis and develop treatment and surveillance plans.[6] The seventh edition of the AJCC staging system has incorporated several histologic features of the primary tumor (tumor thickness, mitotic rate, and ulceration), regional and distant metastasis, which have all been shown to be independent predictors of survival.[6]

Survival Related to Localized Melanoma (Stages I and II)

Breslow[7] first described the depth of tumor invasion correlating with patient outcomes. Thin melanomas (<0.76 mm thickness) were low-risk lesions, seldom metastasized, and were considered prognostically favorable; thick melanomas (>4 mm) had a high risk of recurrence or metastasis, and an unfavorable prognosis. The AJCC considers Breslow thickness as the most important prognostic factor of survival in localized melanoma. Increased primary tumor thickness was associated with a significant decrease in 5- and 10-year survival rates ($P<.0001$). The 10-year survival rates for each T-stage were 92% for T1 ($\leq$1.0 mm thickness), 80% for T2 (1.01–2.0 mm), 63% for T3 (2.01–4.0 mm), and 50% for T4 melanomas (>4.0 mm).[6]

New to the seventh edition AJCC guidelines, the primary tumor's mitotic rate is considered the second most powerful prognostic factor in localized melanoma survival, replacing the Clark level of invasion. The mitotic rate reflects the tumor's proliferation in the vertical growth phase and is defined as the number of mitotic figures counted over an area of 1 mm^2.[8] Tumors with increased mitoses over 1/mm^2 were correlated with worse survival rates ($P<.0001$).[6] The 10-year survival rate for tumors with 0 mitosis/mm^2 was 93% compared with 48% for tumors with at least 20 mitoses/mm^2. As expected, thicker or ulcerated tumors were associated with higher mitotic rates.[9]

The third most powerful survival predictor is the presence of ulceration of the primary tumor. The incidence of ulceration increases as tumor thickness increases.[10] The survival rate of patients with ulcerated tumors was comparable with the rate of the next highest category of a nonulcerated melanoma with increased thickness.[10]

Survival Related to Regional Metastasis (Stage III)

Cox multivariate analysis of the SEER database showed that the total number of nodal metastases, tumor burden of the metastatic deposits (micro- vs macrometastasis), presence of primary tumor ulceration, and Breslow thickness ($P<.001$)[6] were all independent predictors of survival in stage III disease or lymph node-positive melanomas. Survival decreased with increasing nodal involvement (1, 2–3, or 4+ regional nodes), and patients with regional nodal metastasis detected on physical examination (macrometastases) had significantly decreased survival compared with nonpalpable metastatic nodes (**Table 1**).[10] Unlike breast cancer, evaluation of the sentinel lymph node (SLN) for melanoma requires immunohistochemical staining. The AJCC defines micrometastasis as the presence of cells staining positive for 1 melanoma-associated marker (ie, S-100, Melan-A/MART1, HMB-45) and evidence of malignant morphology on hematoxylin and eosin staining.[6,11] Similar to the prognosis for stages I and II, the presence of primary tumor ulceration and increased thickness were associated with lower survival rates.

Survival Related to Distant Metastasis (Stage IV)

Patients with stage IV disease, who have distant metastases, have poor overall survival; however, the specific site of metastasis and serum lactate dehydrogenase (LDH) level can help stratify patients by prognosis and for enrollment into clinical trials. The 1-year survival rate differs depending on the metastatic site: 62% for metastasis to the skin, subcutaneous tissue, or distant lymph nodes (M1a); 53% for pulmonary metastasis (M1b); and 33% for other visceral sites (M1c).[6] Elevated serum LDH levels, in combination with distant metastasis to any site, upstages the patient's classification to M1c, which has the worst prognosis.

Additional Prognostic Survival Factors

Although not identified as independent prognostic factors in the AJCC staging and classification guidelines, several additional risk factors have been reported to be associated with melanoma survival. Female patients seem to have a survival advantage with CM; more men die of the disease than women in the United States (4.1 vs 1.7 deaths per 100,000 persons).[1] In a German study, the gender-associated advantage was lost by the age of 60.[12] Review of the AJCC Melanoma Database and the Sunbelt Melanoma Trial revealed that increasing age correlates with worse prognosis and a decline in survival.[10,13] Garbe and colleagues[14] evaluated the relationship between the primary CM's anatomic site and survival rates. Melanomas located in TANS regions (thorax, upper arm, neck, and scalp) had a less favorable prognosis than those

Table 1
Five-year survival rates for stage III patients with micrometastases versus macrometastases

Number of Positive Nodes	Microscopic + Nodes Survival		Macroscopic + Nodes Survival		
	% ± SE	No.	% ± SE	No.	P^a
1	61 ± 2.8	469	46 ± 3.6	220	<.0001
2	56 ± 4.6	172	37 ± 4.4	139	<.0001
3	56 ± 8.5	69	27 ± 6.0	63	<.001
4	36 ± 8.7	40	24 ± 4.4	106	.1034
>4	35 ± 8.7	73	24 ± 3.5	175	.0011

[a] P value based on the comparison of survival curves using the log-rank test.
Table reproduced with permission from Balch CM, Soong SJ, Gershenwald JE, et al. Prognostic factors analysis of 17,600 melanoma patients: validation of the American Joint Committee on Cancer melanoma staging system. J Clin Oncol 2001;19:3622–34.

located on the lower trunk, thigh, lower leg, foot, lower arms, hands, and face. CMs are more common in fair-skinned races; yet, African Americans, who have an overall lower incidence of melanoma, have a lower 10-year survival rate and higher risk of recurrence after surgical treatment than Caucasians and other races with a comparable stage of disease.[15] Lastly, several other tumor-related factors discussed in the literature may have prognostic value and require future studies: route of invasion (local spread vs lymphatic, hematogenous, perivascular, or distant metastasis), tumor-infiltrating lymphocytes, tumor regression, mutations in molecular markers (N-RAS, Raf, c-Kit, G proteins), alterations in cell-signaling pathways (MAPK, Akt/PI3K, cell cycle, and p53-regulated cell death), and serum markers like S100 and melanoma-inhibiting activity (MIA), a protein secreted by melanoma cells.[11] However, their value remains controversial, and further studies are needed to determine clinical utility.

On-line Melanoma Prognosis Calculators

On-line computer models have been developed to determine a melanoma patient's prognosis based on the AJCC guidelines (www.melanomaprognosis.org).[16] Callender and colleagues[17] improved the prognostic accuracy of the computer model by incorporating sentinel lymph node biopsy (SLNB) results (melanomacalculator.com); they validated their prognostic model using known data from 1001 patients and showed a concordance correlation coefficient (CCC) of 0.984 compared with the AJCC model CCC of 0.784.[17] These computer calculators may be useful tools for physicians to develop individualized care plans and facilitate patient education.

MELANOMA SURVEILLANCE

Despite the variability in recommended melanoma surveillance practice patterns, the purpose is universally identical: early detection of recurrent disease or a new second primary melanoma. Surveillance includes patient education with instructions for self-examination, reassurance, promotion of patient well-being, and monitoring the patient for the development of adverse effects or toxicity due to previous therapies. When recurrent or new lesions are recognized early, appropriate treatment can be initiated expediently, which is believed to improve overall survival outcomes.[18]

Surveillance can be the responsibility of many types of health care providers: primary care physicians (PCPs), nurse practitioners, physician assistants, dermatologists, oncologists, general and plastic surgeons, and a multidisciplinary team for more advanced cases.[19] Also, patient preference and access to care influence who provides surveillance care. McKenna and colleagues[20] performed a retrospective observational study of melanoma surveillance provided by dermatologists, PCPs, and surgical specialists; they found that patients followed by dermatologists had better overall survival, disease-free survival, and recurrence-free survival at 5 years. However, these results may be due to selection bias, because patients treated by dermatologists often had thinner melanomas with better prognostic features.

Most primary melanomas, as well as their recurrences, are first detected by the patient and/or family member, rather than a physician. Recurrences are often identified within the first 2 years after primary tumor diagnosis.[21–23] A recent retrospective study by Salama and colleagues[24] showed that among 11,615 patients originally diagnosed with stage I and II melanomas, the overall risk of initial recurrence peaked at 12 months. They found that for this population, recurrence involving the skin, both local and distant, as well as the regional nodal basin, peaked at 8 months, whereas pulmonary and distant metastatic recurrence peaked at 24 months. Once recurrence was found, the interval to discovery of a second recurrence shortened to 6 months, and the interval to discovery of a third recurrence was further shortened to 2.6 months.[24]

Approximately 1% to 8% of melanoma survivors will develop a second primary melanoma in their lifetime, which is often thinner than the first primary.[25] Physicians, more often than patients, detect the second primary melanoma. The literature is controversial regarding the specific time frame for subsequent melanoma development, and therefore so are the recommendations for the optimal duration of follow-up.[26] Some have reported that the second primary melanoma develops within the first few months to 2 years after initial diagnosis, while others have found that 40% of new primary melanomas were detected more than 7 years later.[22]

Variation in Follow-up Practices

Despite the controversies, some consensus exists among surveillance practices; initial follow-up frequency should be increased in patients with higher AJCC stages of melanoma, and follow-up visits can be less frequent as the patient remains disease-free over time.[19] Also, it is important to note that most studies analyzing follow-up patterns are retrospective in nature. Cromwell and colleagues[25] recently performed a systemic review of published surveillance strategies from 1970 to 2011; they found significant variation in follow-up relative to disease state, country of origin, and physician specialty. The greatest variation in surveillance frequency was noted in stage I patients, which ranged from 1 to 6 visits per year for the first 2 years of treatment, and with regard to the use of routine diagnostic imaging and laboratory evaluations. Universal agreement was reached for all patients to perform self-examinations and to decrease visits to annual surveillance after 5 years of disease-free follow-up.[25]

Turner and colleagues[27] developed a prognostic model to compare the differences in diagnostic detection of recurrences or a new primary for patients undergoing a more frequent (every 3 to 6 months for 5 years followed by annual visits for 5 years) versus a less frequent monitoring strategy (every 4 to 12 months for 2 to 3 years followed by annual visits through 10 years). They found that the less frequent schedule would only delay a diagnosis of recurrence or new primary melanomas for 44.9 and 9.6 patients per 1000 population, respectively, with a time delay of a little over 2 months. They also found the risk of recurrence was greatest in the first year of follow-up, whereas the risk of new primary was constant throughout the 10-year period. The duration of follow-up continues to be debated, and ranges from years to a lifetime of surveillance. **Table 2** compares surveillance recommendations by the National Comprehensive Cancer Network® (NCCN®) and other organizations with published guidelines.[19,25,28]

NCCN Clinical Practice Guidelines in Oncology (NCCN Guidelines®) for Melanoma: Follow-up

The NCCN Guidelines® for Melanoma, Version 3.2014, are an up-to-date set of evidence-based clinical care guidelines established by experts from 25 major cancer centers across the United States. Algorithms for suggested follow-up are based on the clinical/pathologic AJCC stage of disease.[26] For stage 0 (*in situ*) disease, the NCCN® recommends "common follow-up recommendations for all patients," including a minimum of annual skin examinations for life accompanied by patient education on skin and lymph node self-examinations. For patients with stage IA-IIA with no evidence of disease (NED), a history and physical examination should be performed every 6 to 12 months for 5 years, after which annual visits are sufficient. The surveillance schedule of stage IIB-IV patients with NED should include a more

Table 2
Summary of melanoma surveillance guidelines by country

AJCC Staging	Australia/ New Zealand[49]	Canada (BCCA, AHS)[50,51]	Europe (ESMO)[52]	Germany (S3 Guidelines)[53]	United Kingdom (BAD, BAPRAS)[54]	United States (NCCN)[26]	Switzerland[55]
Recommended Number of Visits per Year (Includes ROS and History and Physical Examination)							
Stage 0	1	1	Number consensus	—	0	1	—
Stage I							
Years 1–2	2	1–2	No consensus	2–4	2–4	1–2	2–4
Year 3	2	1–2		2–4	2–4	1–2	2–4
Year 4–5	2	1		1–2	2	1–2	1–2
Year >5	1	1		1–2, up to 10 y	—	1	1–2, up to 10 y
Stage II							
Years 1–2	3–4	2–4	No consensus	4	4	2–4	4
Year 3	3–4	2		4	4	1–4	4
Year 4–5	3–4	1–2		2–4	2	1–4	2–4
Year >5	1	1		1–2 up to 10 y	—	1	1–2, up to 10 y
Stage III-IV							
Years 1–2	3–4	2–4	No consensus	4	4	2–4	4
Year 3	3–4	2–4		4	4	1–4	2
Year 4–5	3–4	1–3		4	2	1–4	2
Year >5	1	1		2, up to 10 y	1, up to 10 y	1	—
Recommended Self-Examinations							
	Yes	Yes	Yes	Yes	Yes	Yes	Yes

Routine Diagnostic Testing and Frequency (Number of Times Per Year)

Stage							
Stage 0	No	No	—	—	No	No	—
Stage I	No	No	—	LNS for stage ≥1B (2)	No	No	No
Stage II	LNS (3–4)	No	—	LNS for stage ≥IIC (2–4); CT (2)	No	Consider brain MRI, chest radiograph, CT, or PET/CT for stage ≥IIB[a]	LNS, CT, MRI, PET, or PET/CT for stage ≥IIC (1–2)
Stage III	LNS (3–4)	No	Consider LNS, CT, or PET/CT	LNS (2–4); CT (2)	Based on clinical need	Consider brain MRI, chest radiograph, CT, or PET/CT[a]	LNS, CT, MRI, PET, or PET/CT (1–2)
Stage IV	LNS (3–4)	No	Consider LNS, CT, or PET/CT	LNS (2–4); CT (2)	Based on clinical need	Consider brain MRI, chest radiograph, CT, or PET/CT[a]	Individualize care
Symptom Initiated	—	Chest radiograph, CT	—	—	LNS, CT, OR PET/CT	Consider chest radiograph, CT, PET/CT, or MRI	—

Routine Laboratory Tests and Frequency (Number of Times Per Year)

	No	No	No	S-100 for stage ≥IB (2–4)	LDH for stage IV	No	S-100 (1–2)

Abbreviations: AHS, Alberta Health Services; BAD, British Association of Dermatologists; BAPRAS, British Association of Plastic, Reconstructive, and Aesthetic Surgeons; BCCA, British Columbia Cancer Agency; ESMO, European Society for Medical Oncology; LDH, lactate dehydrogenase; LNS, lymph node sonography; MRI, magnetic resonance imaging; NCCN, National Comprehensive Cancer Network; ROS, review of systems.

[a] Category 2B recommendation; routine imaging not recommended after first 5 years.

frequent interval of visits, which can be lengthened over time as the chance of recurrence decreases: history and physical examination every 3 to 6 months for 2 years, every 3 to 12 months for 3 years, and annually thereafter. Also, within this 5-year time period after the diagnosis of a primary melanoma, physicians should consider incorporating radiologic imaging (computed tomography [CT], positron emission tomography [PET], and/or magnetic resonance imaging [MRI]) every 4 to 12 months for metastatic surveillance.[26]

Tailoring Surveillance Schedules to Individual Patient Needs

An individual patient's surveillance strategy must account for multiple factors: benefit in outcome improvement, clinical relapse risk profile, coordination of shared care in follow-up, patient's preference, psychosocial needs, access to a support system, and cost-effectiveness of surveillance intensity.[29] A thorough risk profile assessment includes review of a patient's family history of melanoma; presence, extent, and quantity of dysplastic nevi; skin phenotype; risk of nodal recurrence, whether the patient elected for a complete lymphadenectomy (CLND) after a positive SLNB; and history of ultraviolet exposure and skin cancer prevention behavior.[26,30] The practitioner must also take into account how the schedule affects patient convenience, travel time, cost burden, and patient satisfaction, because all of these factors will directly influence patient compliance. Standard follow-up visits must include patient education, which involves the review of surveillance strategies, prognosis, and counseling on disease prevention.

History and physical examination are among the best screening tools for detection of recurrence or new primary CMs.[22,31] At each visit, the practitioner should ask about new or changing cutaneous or subcutaneous lesions, masses, or pain. The review of systems should inquire about the presence of constitutional symptoms like weight loss, neurologic changes, pain, or gastrointestinal or pulmonary complaints, all of which are clues for metastatic disease. The physical examination must include a complete head-to-toe skin examination of sun-exposed and non-sun-exposed sites, including the scalp, conjunctiva, oral mucosa, nails, palms, soles, interdigital web spaces, and the genitalia/perianal area.[30] A thorough lymph node examination should be performed, directing attention toward primary echelon nodes and interval nodes. These practices enable early identification of local/regional/in-transit recurrence or the development of new primary lesions.

Patient Education and Risk Factor Modification

Patients should be instructed on how to perform skin self-examinations (SSEs) and lymph node examinations; yet, studies have shown that most melanoma survivors neither consistently nor comprehensively conduct SSEs.[32] These cost-effective SSEs should be conducted on all skin surfaces in a well-lit area, monthly. If patients have multiple dysplastic nevi, baseline digital photography of lesions can be employed to improve the sensitivity of SSE detecting new lesions.[33] When patients identify new or changing lesions that last more than 2 weeks, they should be advised to report the changes to the practitioner overseeing their surveillance; the 2-week window is suggested, because most acute inflammatory or ecchymotic lesions will resolve within this time frame.[34]

Ultraviolet radiation exposure is a well-established modifiable risk factor; however, studies have shown that although the knowledge about the impact of sun-related behaviors and practice are improved in melanoma patients, there remains an unchanged attitude toward the "healthy" appearance of tans.[35] Recommended sun behavior counseling should include: using sun protection (sunscreen and protective clothing), reducing ambient and recreational sun exposure, seeking shade when possible, and avoiding sunburns and tanning bed usage.[36]

Evaluation of Psychosocial Distress and Coping Mechanisms

The psychosocial impact of melanoma can be profound. Anxiety and depression are the most commonly reported emotions experienced by melanoma patients, which can be manifested in a variety of ways: delay in seeking medical care, poor compliance, a lower quality of life (QoL), increased medical visits and cost, and reduced participation in surveillance programs.[37,38] Validated instruments available for QoL assessment include the Functional Assessment of Cancer Therapy Scale–Melanoma questionnaire[39] and the Malignant Melanoma Module, which is currently being updated in collaboration with the European Organization for Research and Treatment of Cancer Quality of Life Group.[40,41]

Reassessment of the psychosocial impact of melanoma is necessary, as patients experience different reactions to their disease over the course of survivorship: problems moving past the cancer diagnosis, feelings of abandonment as visits become less frequent over time, a sense of watchful waiting for recurrence, difficulty living with on-going physical limitations and a distorted body image after surgery, and struggling to find positive meaning in life.[42] Coping mechanisms of patients can significantly impact QoL; more functional styles like problem-focused coping should be promoted over avoidance or denial.[43] In a randomized controlled trial of melanoma patients during various stages of survivorship, Fawzy and colleagues[44] found that psychiatric interventions incorporating education, stress management, enhancement of coping skills, and psychological support were associated with greater disease-free intervals and survival than the control group.

Some patients think that regular clinic visits evoke a sense of safety and reassurance; however, others may perceive frequent follow-up as a source of anxiety, fear, and a repeated reminder of the possibility of cancer recurrence and mortality. The physician can help develop a tailored supportive care program in the form of educational techniques, behavioral or skill training, social support, and psychotherapy; referrals to psychologists, counselors, or group programs may also benefit the patient or caregiver.[42] Patient satisfaction with follow-up visits is improved with practitioner accessibility, and continuity of care provides patients with a sense of confidence in the clinical care provided.[37] Lastly, education and support can help alleviate the burden of disease on caregivers.

DIAGNOSIS AND MANAGEMENT OF MELANOMA RECURRENCE

Melanoma recurrence can be divided into several categories: local, in-transit/satellite, regional, or distant. Moreover, local recurrence is subdivided into local scar and true local recurrence. The first recurrence of melanoma most often involves the regional lymph nodes (50%), and less commonly, local/in-transit/satellite disease (20%), and distant metastasis (30%)[25,34]; these statistics are likely to change as SLNBs with completion nodal basin dissection for positive nodal disease are now utilized routinely, identifying micrometastasis earlier.

Local Scar Recurrence

Local scar recurrence is caused by persistent disease and is defined by the presence of *in situ* and/or a radial growth phase. Local recurrence occurs within a 2 cm radius of the scar or skin graft. The work-up of melanoma recurrence should parallel how primary tumors are managed.[26] Local scar recurrence is confirmed by biopsy/fine needle aspiration (FNA), and its management is comparable to that of primary tumors with the same stage. Wide local re-excision should be performed and lymphatic mapping/SLNB or adjuvant therapy may be considered.

Local, Satellite, and In-transit Recurrence

True local recurrence develops after an initial adequate primary tumor excision, and its incidence increases with primary melanoma thickness and ulceration.[45] Local recurrence commonly develops from dermal lymphatic disease in close proximity to the scar, whereas satellite and in-transit disease results from endolymphatic spread. Locoregional disease manifests as cutaneous or subcutaneous nodules between the primary tumor site and the regional nodal basin, and should be considered recurrence until proven otherwise.[26,45] These tumors may or may not be palpable, and when visible, they are often pink or flesh colored rather than hyperpigmented like a traditional melanoma tumor.

Local, satellite, or in-transit lesions should be confirmed pathologically by biopsy or cytology from FNA. Chest radiographs, CT scan, PET scan, MRI, or lymph node ultrasonography may be used to investigate signs and symptoms concerning for metastasis. The standard of care for resectable locoregional recurrence is surgical resection with negative margins. Depending on the size and anatomic location of the tumor, skin grafting or flap closure may be employed for wound coverage.

Additional treatment options for locoregional disease include enrollment in a clinical trial, nonsurgical local therapies like intralesional injections of the bacillus Calmette-Guérin (BCG) or granulocyte–macrophage colony stimulating factor, phototherapy with a pulsed dye or carbon dioxide laser, topical agents like imiquimod (immunomodulator and toll-like receptor agonist), diphencyprone (a contact sensitizer for superficial dermal lesions), regional therapies like isolated limb infusion (ILI)/hyperthermic isolated limb perfusion (HILP) with melphalan, systemic therapies like interferon alpha (IFN-α) or interleukin-2 (IL-2), electrochemotherapy (which involves the delivery of high-intensity electrical pulses to cause cell membrane poration and increase chemotherapeutic delivery), and palliative radiation therapy for unresectable disease.[26,31,46] Adjuvant therapeutic options for locoregional recurrence include joining a clinical trial, observation, or initiation of high-dose IFN-α therapy.

Regional Recurrence

Regional recurrence directly involves the lymph nodes. Romano and colleagues[47] found that the first recurrence among stage III patients was more often systemic (51%) rather than local/in-transit (28%) or regional (21%). This is speculated to be occult nodal micrometastasis that, over time, develops into palpable nodal metastasis and spreads to distant sites.[34] Recurrent regional malignancies are more likely to develop after unfavorable primary tumor characteristics (increased Breslow thickness, mitoses, ulceration), lesions of the head and neck, and an initially (false) negative SLNB.[46]

Regional recurrence should be confirmed pathologically by FNA (preferred) or lymph node biopsy, and work-up is similar to that of primary stage III tumors. Patients without previous nodal dissection or history of an incomplete resection should undergo CLND.[26] If the patient had a prior CLND, the recurrence should be excised to negative margins. As shown in the international Multicenter Selective Lymphadenectomy Trial (MSLT-1), delayed CLND is a morbid procedure significantly associated chronic lymphedema.[48] Treatment options for unresectable locoregional or systemic disease include enrollment in a clinical trial, radiation therapy, systemic therapy, IFN-α, or supportive care.

Metastatic Recurrence

Lastly, the presentation of distant recurrence can vary, manifesting as a single lesion or as multifocal disease. The most common sites of metastasis are brain, lung, and liver; less common sites include the skin, distant lymph nodes, bone, adrenal glands, or gastrointestinal tract.[31,34]

The work-up and treatment of distant metastatic disease are similar to that of primary stage IV melanoma. Pathologic diagnosis is required, preferably by FNA rather than biopsy. The extent of baseline disease should be characterized with serum LDH levels and CT of the chest/abdomen/pelvis, MRI, and/or PET scan. Treatment options depend on whether the distant metastasis is limited and resectable versus disseminated and unresectable.[26]

If feasible, surgical resection of solitary metastatic lesions is recommended, but patients can be offered the alternatives of observation or systemic therapy followed by repeat scans to measure disease progression. Management options for patients with disseminated disease include systemic therapy, clinical trial, palliative resection and/or radiation therapy for symptomatic patients, or supportive care. Current preferred systemic therapy regimens include ipilimumab, vemurafenib for melanomas with BRAF mutations, and high-dose IL-2.[26] Additional options include dacarbazine and/or temozolomide, imatinib for tumors with c-KIT mutations, cisplatin and vinblastine with or without IL-2, IFN-α, and paclitaxel alone or in combination with carboplatin.[26] As with any systemic therapy, patients should be monitored closely for adverse effects and toxicity. When patients have brain metastasis, surgical intervention and/or radiation is recommended to minimize or delay central nervous system morbidity, and such therapies include stereotactic radiosurgery or whole-brain radiotherapy.

SUMMARY

The incidence of melanoma continues to rise while mortality rates remain stable, resulting in a growing population of melanoma survivors. The development of surveillance strategies must be tailored to each individual patient, taking into consideration tumor stage, prognosis relative to the initial primary tumor characteristics, and risk factors for recurrence or a second primary tumor. General agreement exists regarding frequent follow-up visits for advanced stages of melanoma initially, and as the patient's disease-free interval increases, visits can be less frequent. Critical components of each follow-up visit include history and physical examination, reinforcement of skin and lymph node self-examination, sun behavior counseling, evaluation of patient well-being, and development of coping skills.

Surgical resection with negative margins is the treatment of choice for operable local, satellite, and in-transit regional recurrence; additional therapeutic options for locoregional recurrence vary from intralesional injections of BCG to regional ILI/HILP, immunomodulators, systemic therapies, and enrollment in clinical trials. Regional nodal recurrence should be excised and CLND performed if not completed previously. Management of metastatic recurrence depends on whether distant metastasis is limited or disseminated. For complex cases, melanoma survivorship may best be managed by a multidisciplinary team of specialists, each of whom is expert in his or her respective field.

REFERENCES

1. Howlader N, Noone AM, Krapcho M, et al. Surveillance, Epidemiology, and End Results (SEER) cancer statistics review, 1975–2010. Available at: http://seer.cancer.gov/csr/1975_2010/. Accessed March 6, 2014.
2. MacKie RM, Hauschild A, Eggermont AM. Epidemiology of invasive cutaneous melanoma. Ann Oncol 2009;20(Suppl 6):vi1–7.

3. Garbe C, Leiter U. Melanoma epidemiology and trends. Clin Dermatol 2009;27: 3–9.

4. Yang GB, Barnholtz-Sloan JS, Chen Y, et al. Risk and survival of cutaneous melanoma diagnosed subsequent to a previous cancer. Arch Dermatol 2011;147: 1395–402.

5. Freedman DM, Miller BA, Tucker MA. New malignancies following melanoma of the skin, eye melanoma, and non-melanoma eye cancer. In: Curtis RE, Freedman DM, Ron E, et al, editors. New malignancies among cancer survivors: SEER cancer registries, 1973–2000. Bethesda (MD): National Cancer Institute; 2006. p. 339–62.

6. Balch CM, Gershenwald JE, Soong SJ, et al. Final version of 2009 AJCC melanoma staging and classification. J Clin Oncol 2009;27:6199–206.

7. Breslow A. Thickness, cross-sectional areas and depth of invasion in the prognosis of cutaneous melanoma. Ann Surg 1970;172:902–8.

8. Mervic L. Prognostic factors in patients with localized primary cutaneous melanoma. Acta Dermatovenerol Alp Pannonica Adriat 2012;21:27–31.

9. Thompson JF, Soong SJ, Balch CM, et al. Prognostic significance of mitotic rate in localized primary cutaneous melanoma: an analysis of patients in the multi-institutional American Joint Committee on Cancer melanoma staging database. J Clin Oncol 2011;29:2199–205.

10. Balch CM, Soong SJ, Gershenwald JE, et al. Prognostic factors analysis of 17,600 melanoma patients: validation of the American Joint Committee on Cancer melanoma staging system. J Clin Oncol 2001;19:3622–34.

11. Fernandez-Flores A. Prognostic factors for melanoma progression and metastasis: from hematoxylin–eosin to genetics. Rom J Morphol Embryol 2012;53:449–59.

12. Mervic L, Leiter U, Meier F, et al. Sex differences in survival of cutaneous melanoma are age dependent: an analysis of 7338 patients. Melanoma Res 2011;21: 244–52.

13. Chao C, Martin RC 2nd, Ross MI, et al. Correlation between prognostic factors and increasing age in melanoma. Ann Surg Oncol 2004;11:259–64.

14. Garbe C, Buttner P, Bertz J, et al. Primary cutaneous melanoma. Prognostic classification of anatomic location. Cancer 1995;75:2492–8.

15. Collins KK, Fields RC, Baptiste D, et al. Racial differences in survival after surgical treatment for melanoma. Ann Surg Oncol 2011;18:2925–36.

16. Soong SJ, Ding S, Coit DG, et al. Individualized melanoma patient outcome prediction tools. Developed based on the American Joint Committee on Cancer Melanoma Database. Available at: www.melanomaprognosis.org. Accessed March 16, 2014.

17. Callender GG, Gershenwald JE, Egger ME, et al. A novel and accurate computer model of melanoma prognosis for patients staged by sentinel lymph node biopsy: comparison with the American Joint Committee on Cancer model. J Am Coll Surg 2012;214:608–19.

18. Garbe C, Paul A, Kohler-Spath H, et al. Prospective evaluation of a follow-up schedule in cutaneous melanoma patients: recommendations for an effective follow-up strategy. J Clin Oncol 2003;21:520–9.

19. Trotter SC, Sroa N, Winkelmann RR, et al. A global review of melanoma follow-up guidelines. J Clin Aesthet Dermatol 2013;6:18–26.

20. McKenna DB, Marioni JC, Lee RJ, et al. A comparison of dermatologists', surgeons' and general practitioners' surgical management of cutaneous melanoma. Br J Dermatol 2004;151:636–44.

21. Epstein DS, Lange JR, Gruber SB, et al. Is physician detection associated with thinner melanomas? JAMA 1999;281:640–3.

22. Francken AB, Bastiaannet E, Hoekstra HJ. Follow-up in patients with localised primary cutaneous melanoma. Lancet Oncol 2005;6:608–21.

23. Francken AB, Shaw HM, Accortt NA, et al. Detection of first relapse in cutaneous melanoma patients: implications for the formulation of evidence-based follow-up guidelines. Ann Surg Oncol 2007;14:1924–33.

24. Salama AK, de Rosa N, Scheri RP, et al. Hazard-rate analysis and patterns of recurrence in early stage melanoma: moving towards a rationally designed surveillance strategy. PLoS One 2013;8:e57665.

25. Cromwell KD, Ross MI, Xing Y, et al. Variability in melanoma post-treatment surveillance practices by country and physician specialty: a systematic review. Melanoma Res 2012;22:376–85.

26. Coit DG, Thompson JA, Andtbacka R, et al. NCCN clinical practice guidelines in oncology (NCCN guidelines®) for melanoma (version 3.2014). Available at: http://www.nccn.org/professionals/physician_gls/f_guidelines.asp. Accessed March 9, 2014.

27. Turner RM, Bell KJ, Morton RL, et al. Optimizing the frequency of follow-up visits for patients treated for localized primary cutaneous melanoma. J Clin Oncol 2011;29:4641–6.

28. Fong ZV, Tanabe KK. Comparison of melanoma guidelines in the U.S.A., Canada, Europe, Australia and New Zealand: a critical appraisal and comprehensive review. Br J Dermatol 2014;170:20–30.

29. Rychetnik L, McCaffery K, Morton RL, et al. Follow-up of early stage melanoma: specialist clinician perspectives on the functions of follow-up and implications for extending follow-up intervals. J Surg Oncol 2013;107:463–8.

30. Brown MD. Office management of melanoma patients. Semin Cutan Med Surg 2010;29:232–7.

31. Dunki-Jacobs EM, Callender GG, McMasters KM. Current management of melanoma. Curr Probl Surg 2013;50:351–82.

32. Mujumdar UJ, Hay JL, Monroe-Hinds YC, et al. Sun protection and skin self-examination in melanoma survivors. Psychooncology 2009;18:1106–15.

33. Oliveria SA, Chau D, Christos PJ, et al. Diagnostic accuracy of patients in performing skin self-examination and the impact of photography. Arch Dermatol 2004;140:57–62.

34. Benvenuto-Andrade C, Oseitutu A, Agero AL, et al. Cutaneous melanoma: surveillance of patients for recurrence and new primary melanomas. Dermatol Ther 2005;18:423–35.

35. Lee TK, Brazier AS, Shoveller JA, et al. Sun-related behavior after a diagnosis of cutaneous malignant melanoma. Melanoma Res 2007;17:51–5.

36. Geller AC, O'Riordan DL, Oliveria SA, et al. Overcoming obstacles to skin cancer examinations and prevention counseling for high-risk patients: results of a national survey of primary care physicians. J Am Board Fam Pract 2004;17:416–23.

37. McLoone JK, Watts KJ, Menzies SW, et al. Melanoma survivors at high risk of developing new primary disease: a qualitative examination of the factors that contribute to patient satisfaction with clinical care. Psychooncology 2013;22:1994–2000.

38. Kasparian NA. Psychological stress and melanoma: are we meeting our patients' psychological needs? Clin Dermatol 2013;31:41–6.

39. Cella DF, Tulsky DS, Gray G, et al. The Functional Assessment of Cancer Therapy scale: development and validation of the general measure. J Clin Oncol 1993;11:570–9.

40. Sigurdardottir V, Bolund C, Brandberg Y, et al. The impact of generalized malignant melanoma on quality of life evaluated by the EORTC questionnaire technique. Qual Life Res 1993;2:193–203.

41. Winstanley JB, White EG, Boyle FM, et al. What are the pertinent quality-of-life issues for melanoma cancer patients? Aiming for the development of a new module to accompany the EORTC core questionnaire. Melanoma Res 2013; 23:167–74.

42. Tan JD, Butow PN, Boyle FM, et al. A qualitative assessment of psychosocial impact, coping and adjustment in high-risk melanoma patients and caregivers. Melanoma Res 2014;24:252–60.

43. Vurnek M, Buljan M, Situm M. Psychological status and coping with illness in patients with malignant melanoma. Coll Antropol 2007;31(Suppl 1):53–6.

44. Fawzy FI, Fawzy NW, Hyun CS, et al. Malignant melanoma. Effects of an early structured psychiatric intervention, coping, and affective state on recurrence and survival 6 years later. Arch Gen Psychiatry 1993;50:681–9.

45. Levine SM, Shapiro RL. Surgical treatment of malignant melanoma: practical guidelines. Dermatol Clin 2012;30:487–501.

46. Squires MH 3rd, Delman KA. Current treatment of locoregional recurrence of melanoma. Curr Oncol Rep 2013;15:465–72.

47. Romano E, Scordo M, Dusza SW, et al. Site and timing of first relapse in stage III melanoma patients: implications for follow-up guidelines. J Clin Oncol 2010;28: 3042–7.

48. Morton DL. Overview and update of the phase III Multicenter Selective Lymphadenectomy Trials (MSLT-I and MSLT-II) in melanoma. Clin Exp Metastasis 2012; 29:699–706.

49. Australian Cancer Network Melanoma Guidelines Revision Working Party. Clinical practice guidelines for the management of melanoma in Australia and New Zealand. Cancer Council Australia and Australian Cancer Network, Sydney and New Zealand Guidelines Group. Available at: https://www.nhmrc.gov.au/guidelines/publications/cp111. Accessed March 6, 2014.

50. British Columbia Cancer Agency. Melanoma follow-up. Available at: http://www.bccancer.bc.ca/HPI/CancerManagementGuidelines/Skin/Melanoma/ManagementPolicies/Follow-up.htm. Accessed March 6, 2014.

51. Alberta Cutaneous Tumor Team. Referral and follow-up surveillance of cutaneous melanoma. Available at: http://www.albertahealthservices.ca/hp/if-hp-cancer-guide-cu001-followup-surveillance.pdf. Accessed March 6, 2014.

52. Dummer R, Hauschild A, Guggenheim M, et al. Cutaneous melanoma: ESMO clinical practice guidelines for diagnosis, treatment and follow-up. Ann Oncol 2012;23(Suppl 7):vii86–91.

53. Pflugfelder A, Kochs C, Blum A, et al. S3-guideline "diagnosis, therapy and follow-up of melanoma"—short version. J Dtsch Dermatol Ges 2013;11:563–602.

54. Marsden JR, Newton-Bishop JA, Burrows L, et al. Revised UK guidelines for the management of cutaneous melanoma 2010. J Plast Reconstr Aesthet Surg 2010;63:1401–19.

55. Dummer R, Guggenheim M, Arnold AW, et al. Updated Swiss guidelines for the treatment and follow-up of cutaneous melanoma. Swiss Med Wkly 2011;141: w13320.

Locoregional Therapies in Melanoma

Andrea M. Abbott, MD, MS, Jonathan S. Zager, MD*

KEYWORDS

- Melanoma • Locoregional recurrence • Isolated limb infusion
- Hyperthermic isolated limb perfusion • Intra-tumoral injections

KEY POINTS

- In-transit disease should be approached with a multimodality treatment strategy in mind.
- Resection with the primary goal to remove all disease is the ideal initial strategy.
- Patients with a heavy burden of disease may benefit from regional perfusion.
- Intralesional injection is a well-tolerated method to control locoregional disease and some agents have been shown to have a systemic bystander effect.

SURGICAL RESECTION

When a local, satellite, or in-transit recurrence is suspected, the National Comprehensive Cancer Network (NCCN) guidelines currently recommend fine-needle aspiration or biopsy to confirm diagnosis.[1–4] Once the diagnosis of recurrent disease is confirmed, computed tomography (CT) and/or positron emission tomography/CT (PET) or magnetic resonance imaging (MRI) should be performed for initial staging. The NCCN advocates wide excision with negative margins if the entire extent of disease can be resected and the patient rendered no evidence of disease (NED); this approach might offer the best chance for long-term disease-free survival.[5] The depth of the primary tumor does not affect margin width when treating regionally recurrent disease and in our center we strive to get 1-cm grossly negative radial margins, and a negative deep fascial plane in surgery.[1] In a review of 648 patients with local recurrence from cutaneous melanoma by Dong and colleagues,[6] all patients were initially treated with resection of the local recurrence. After resection, 124 patients (19%) had no further progression, whereas 196 (30%) developed another local recurrence, 178 (27%) developed in-transit disease, and 150 (23%) had distant recurrences. In this series many of the patients who had progression of disease went on to be treated with additional local, intra-arterial perfusion or systemic therapies. Survival was 77.4%

Department of Cutaneous Oncology, Moffitt Cancer Center, 12902 Magnolia Drive, SRB 4.24012, Tampa, FL 33612, USA
* Corresponding author.
E-mail address: jonathan.zager@moffitt.org

Surg Clin N Am 94 (2014) 1003–1015
http://dx.doi.org/10.1016/j.suc.2014.07.004
0039-6109/14/$ – see front matter © 2014 Elsevier Inc. All rights reserved.

surgical.theclinics.com

for patients with no progression of disease after resection of the initial recurrence with a median follow-up of 39 months.[6]

Patients with in-transit disease are at high risk for occult nodal involvement; however, the impact of sentinel lymph node biopsy (SLNB) in this setting has not been fully evaluated.[4] There is no consensus at this time on performance of SLNB in patients who have recurrent locoregional or in-transit disease, regardless of any history of previous SLNB or lymphadenectomy.[4,5] The feasibility of identifying a sentinel lymph node (SLN) in patients with prior SLNB has been established.[7,8] Although some investigators have found a difference in median disease-free survival between patients with positive SLNB compared with patients with negative SLNB with in-transit disease, there was no difference in overall survival.[7] In a study by Yao and colleagues,[7] 30 patients underwent lymphatic mapping and SLNB for recurrent melanoma. Fourteen (47%) patients were found to have positive SLN and 11 (78%) then underwent complete lymph node dissection (CLND). The patients who had positive SLNB had worse median disease-free survival: 16 months (range 1–108 months) compared with 36 months (range 6–132 months) for patients with negative SLNB ($P = .0251$). Beasley and colleagues[8] found a similarly high rate of nodal disease in their study of 33 patients with in-transit melanoma who underwent lymphatic mapping and SLNB. A SLN was identified in 30 cases and 10 (33%) patients had positive nodes. Nine patients then underwent CLND and additional lymph node involvement was found in 4 of these patients (44% non-SLN involvement). In this cohort, 79% (26 of 33) of patients had previously undergone some form of lymph node resection (either SLNB or CLND) in the same lymph node basin as the expected drainage of the in-transit recurrence.

INTRA-ARTERIAL REGIONAL PERFUSION THERAPIES
Hyperthermic Isolated Limb Perfusion

Hyperthermic isolated limb perfusion (HILP) is a method by which an extremity with locoregional or in-transit metastatic melanoma is isolated from systemic circulation and high-dose chemotherapy is administered with limited systemic exposure. First described in 1958 by Creech and colleagues,[9] HILP is performed by directly dissecting and cannulating the major vessels of the root of the extremity and infusing and circulating chemotherapy via a cardiopulmonary bypass machine. The limb vasculature is isolated from systemic circulation with the aid of a tourniquet and collateral vessels are ligated. In the lower extremity femoral or external iliac vessels are used and subclavian or axillary vessels are cannulated for upper extremity disease. The chemotherapy is recirculated for 60 minutes and is then washed out with 2 L of a balanced electrolyte solution. In addition to achieving concentrations 15 to 25 times higher than would be tolerated with systemic chemotherapy, HILP is also performed in the setting of hyperthermia. The limb temperatures reach 39°C to 41°C, which potentially augments the effects of the melphalan-based chemotherapy.[10,11] Flow rates are typically 400 to 600 mL/min and a pump oxygenator is used to oxygenate the perfusate.

The response rates to HILP vary throughout the literature and overall response rates have been reported in the range of 80% to 90% with complete response (CR) rates as high as 60% to 70% (**Table 1**).[10,12–15] The addition of hyperthermia has been shown to have a positive effect on CR.[11] Melphalan is the most common agent used in the United States and melphalan plus tumor necrosis factor alpha (TNF-α) is often used in Europe. The addition of TNF-α has been shown to improve CR in the European literature; however, these results have not been consistently reproducible.[16,17] The American College of Surgeons Oncology Group (ACOSOG) Z0020 trial was a large multicenter trial in the United States in which patients received either melphalan or

Table 1
Summary of response rates from major HILP and isolated limb infusion (ILI) studies

Author, Year	Regional Perfusion Method (HILP or ILI)	Agent Used	Study Population (N)	Response Rates (%)	Toxicity/Adverse Events (%)
Raymond et al,[23] 2011	HILP	Melphalan	N = 77	OR: 81 CR: 55 PR: 26	Grade 1 or 2: 73 Grade ≥3: 27 2 Amputations
Cornett et al,[15] 2006	HILP	Melphalan Melphalan + TNF-α	N = 65 N = 68	OR: 64 melphalan 69 melphalan + TNF-α CR: 25 melphalan 26 melphalan + TNF-α	Grade 4: 12 Melphalan: 4 Melphalan + TNF-α: 16 1 Amputation (grade 5): Melphalan + TNF-α
Noorda et al,[12] 2004	HILP	Melphalan Melphalan + TNF-α	N = 40 N = 90	CR: 45 melphalan 59 melphalan + TNF-α	Grade 1 or 2: Melphalan: 71 Melphalan + TNF-α: 75 Grade 3: Melphalan: 26 Melphalan + TNF-α: 23 Grade 4: Melphalan: 3 Melphalan + TNF-α: 2
Coventry et al,[50] 2014	ILI	Melphalan	N = 131	OR: 63 CR: 27 PR: 36	Grade ≥3: 13 Grade 5: 0
Wong et al,[51] 2013	ILI	Melphalan ± actinomycin D	N = 79	OR: 72 CR: 32 PR: 40	Grade 3: 23 Grade 4: 0 Grade 5: 0
Raymond et al,[23] 2011	ILI	Melphalan ± actinomycin D	N = 148	OR: 43 CR: 30 PR: 13	Grade 1 or 2: 80 Grade ≥3: 20 Grade 5: 0
Beasley et al,[26] 2009	ILI	Melphalan ± actinomycin D	N = 162	OR: 64 CR: 31 PR: 33	Grade ≥3: 36 1 Amputation

Abbreviations: CR, complete response; HILP, hyperthermic isolated limb perfusion; ILI, isolated limb infusion; OR, overall response; PR, partial response; TNF, tumor necrosis factor.

melphalan plus TNF-α. Complete responses of 25% in the melphalan group versus 26% in the melphalan plus TNF-α group were reported at 3 months, with no statistically significant difference seen in either overall response (OR) or CR rates (P = .435 OR, P = .890 CR). The addition of TNF-α was also associated with significantly higher regional toxicity. A 16% grade IV adverse event rate was reported in the melphalan plus TNF-α group versus 4% in the melphalan alone-group (P = .04).[15] Because of the lack of increased efficacy and the increased toxicity from the addition of TNF-α seen in the ACOSOG trial, HILP in the United States is now performed with melphalan alone.

Isolation of the limb during HILP substantially minimizes the risk of systemic toxicity from the high-dose chemotherapy; however, significant morbidity may still occur. Complications may be secondary to the surgical dissection required to isolate the vessels necessary for cannulation, regional toxicity secondary to chemotherapy infusion and/or effects from regional hyperthermia, or systemic effects from leakage of chemotherapy into systemic circulation. The most common morbidity is lymphedema, which has been reported to occur in 12% to 36% of patients.[18] Acute tissue reactions seen after HILP are often classified using the Wieberdink (WBD) grading system, which describes the grading of extremity/regional toxicity. Grade I toxicity is no reaction, grade II is slight erythema or edema, grade III is considerable edema or erythema with some blistering, and grade IV is characterized by extensive epidermolysis or obvious damage to deep tissues. Grade IV toxicities may result in functional impairment or even compartment syndrome requiring fasciotomy. Grade V reactions are severe tissue necrosis or vascular catastrophe that often results in amputation.[19] Compartment syndrome requiring fasciotomy after HILP has been reported in the literature up to 5%.[12,18,20] Grade V WBD toxicity resulting in limb amputation is rare but has been described in certain series in up to 3.3% of cases.[15,18] During the procedure, systemic leakage of the chemotherapy is monitored with a precordial probe used to detect radiolabeled red blood cells in the circuit that may leak into the systemic circulation. Systemic side effects from melphalan such as gastrointestinal disturbance, myelosuppression, or hypotension may develop and the addition of TNF-α has been associated with higher rates of systemic toxicity. The systemic effects of TNF-α include cardiovascular effects such as tachycardia, hypotension, decreased systemic vascular resistance, and increased cardiac output, as well as liver dysfunction.[21] Reduction in the flow rate during HILP has been associated with a reduction in the rate of the chemotherapeutic agent leakage into the systemic circulation.[21]

Isolated Limb Infusion

Isolated limb infusion (ILI) is the less invasive counterpart to HILP. As in HILP, high-dose chemotherapy is administered to the affected limb; however, ILI is a low-flow (typically 80–120 mL/min) perfusion conducted in a hyperthermic, acidotic, and hypoxic environment. Under fluoroscopic guidance 5-French or 6-French high-flow catheters are percutaneously placed into the artery and vein of the uninvolved limb. The catheter tips are advanced into the artery and vein of the involved limb proximal to the extent of disease. Systemic heparinization is administered and warming blankets/liquid gel warming pads are placed on the extremity to expedite the warming process and decrease intraoperative general anesthetic time. An extracorporeal circuit with an external heating source may be used and once circulation is established a pneumatic or Esmarch tourniquet is used to isolate the limb from the systemic circulation. As in HILP, temperature probes closely monitor the subcutaneous and intramuscular tissue temperature with a goal temperature of greater than 37 C before the perfusate is then rapidly infused into the arterial line. The chemotherapy is then recirculated for 30 minutes and, once completed, the limb is flushed via the arterial catheter with isotonic saline until the effluent collected via the venous side is clear.[22]

Complete responses after ILI have been reported to be in the range of 23% to 44% with partial responses rates (PR) reported to be in the range of 27% to 56%.[22–25] In the study by Kroon and colleagues[24] from the Melanoma Institute of Australia, patients who achieved a CR had a longer median duration of response: 24 months, compared with 9 months in patients who only achieved a PR. This same study also found that median disease-specific survival times were significantly longer in those patients who achieved a CR compared with PR (42 months vs 32 months; $P = .04$).

The morbidity associated with ILI is slightly different than that of HILP. The nature of the procedure, percutaneous access versus surgical dissection and direct cannulation, reduces the risks associated with longer operative times and groin or axillary dissections. ILI also has minimal systemic side effects. However, like HILP, ILI has the potential for regional complications. Erythema and edema of the skin with localized inflammation are among the most common side effects.[25] In a multi-institutional study of more than 150 patients, 32% of patients experienced grade 3 or higher WBD toxicity. One patient required an amputation after grade 5 toxicity.[26] Creatinine kinase (CK) levels correlate with a risk of toxicity and the higher the peak level the more likely the patient is to experience severe (grade III or higher) WBD toxicity.[27] Overall, it appears as if ILI is associated with a lower risk of severe, limb-threatening complications and systemic toxicities compared with HILP (**Table 2**).

There is some debate regarding whether ILI or HILP should be used first in the patient with metastatic in-transit melanoma. HILP seems to have better initial OR but the toxicity seems to be much greater than that of ILI. Another potential advantage of ILI as a first approach is that no surgical incisions are made and tissue planes are not disrupted, allowing HILP to be a secondary treatment if the condition recurs after ILI. One scenario in which HILP might be performed rather than ILI is when there are clinically positive nodes and a CLND can be easily done at the same time as HILP, whereas it is not routinely done when ILI is performed. Therefore, a patient with clinically positive nodes may benefit from HILP instead of ILI. However, a node dissection can be performed after an ILI in the same operative setting. It is advisable to perform the node dissection second because of the anticoagulation during an ILI and the risk of bleeding in a fresh CLND basin. Chai and colleagues[28] proposed a treatment algorithm for patients with in-transit disease. The investigators proposed that ILI should

Table 2	
ILI and HILP comparison	
ILI	**HILP**
Low flow rates of 80–120 mL/min	High flow rates of 400–600 mL/min
Normothermic to slightly hyperthermic 37°C–40°C	Hyperthermia >38°C
Minimally invasive, percutaneous introduced catheters	Open, surgical cannulation of the vessels at the root of the extremity
Easy to repeat procedure	Difficult to repeat procedure
Ischemic, anaerobic, acidotic perfusate	Aerobic, oxygenated, mildly acidic perfusate
Melphalan and actinomycin D	Melphalan (±TNF Europe)
Overall responses reported to be as high as 84%, complete responses up to 44%	Overall responses reported to be as high as 90% with complete responses up to 40%–60% (greater with TNF in some studies)

be used for initial regional perfusions, except possibly in the case of high burden of disease. The investigators suggested that HILP be reserved as a salvage procedure for patients who progress rapidly after ILI. Repeat ILI can be attempted in patients who had a good initial response to ILI but relapse. In the Chai and colleagues[28] series, patients who underwent ILI and then had repeat ILI for recurrence had an OR of 40% and a CR of 24%. Patients who underwent HILP after initial ILI treatment had a better OR of 70% and a CR of 50%. This difference in response rates between ILI followed a repeat ILI versus ILI followed by an HILP after recurrence or progression of regional disease was not statistically significant likely due to small numbers in the studies. These findings were similar to those reported by Kroon and colleagues,[29] who studied 48 patients who were treated with repeat ILI for recurrent or progressive disease after an initial ILI treatment. The CR was 23% with an OR of 83% after redo ILI. The median duration of response was 11 months. Repeat ILI was associated with a significantly higher rate of grade 3 and 4 toxicity when compared to the initial ILI. After initial ILI, 14 patients (29%) had a grade 3 toxicity and 1 patient (2%) had grade 4 toxicity; however, after undergoing repeat ILI, 20 patients developed grade 3 toxicity (42%) and 5 patients (10%) had grade 4 toxicity ($P = .03$).

INTRALESIONAL AND TOPICAL THERAPIES
Bacille Calmette-Guerin

Bacille Calmette-Guerin (BCG) is the most recognized intralesional therapy for in-transit metastases. The first report of intralesional injection of BCG was published in 1974 by Morton and colleagues.[30] In that series 90% of cutaneous lesions that were injected showed regression and 17% of those patients also had regression of uninjected (bystander) lesions. A 31% disease-free survival was achieved and sustained for up to 74 months after injection.[30] Additional studies have had mixed results. In one of the largest studies exploring the use of BCG for in-transit melanoma, ECOG 1673, conducted by the Eastern Cooperative Oncology Group (ECOG), patients received either BCG, BCG with dacarbazine, or observation. There was no survival difference among the 3 treatment arms.[31]

The administration of intralesional BCG is time and labor intensive, requiring several treatments until regression of tumor is achieved. The side effects associated with BCG include injection site reaction, seroconversion, and systemic infection. Because of the potentially severe nature of these adverse events and the improved safety profile of newer agents, the use of BCG is declining.

Interleukin-2

Interleukin-2 (IL-2) has been approved for intralesional injection for patients with locally recurrent and in-transit metastases. In a pilot study of 24 patients by Radny and colleagues,[32] a 63% CR was reported and a PR was observed in 21%. This study was conducted in patients who failed surgery, perfusion, radiation, or chemotherapy. In a smaller study of 10 patients with multiple in-transit or subcutaneous nodules, patients were treated with granulocyte macrophage-colony stimulating factor (GM-CSF) initially followed by IL-2 in the case of failure.[33] The combination of GM-CSF and IL-2 resulted in a CR in 6 patients that was sustained for more than 6 months.[33]

The toxicity profile of IL-2 seems to be better than that of BCG. There is a risk of local reactions, but systemic side effects have not been reported. The drawback of this therapy is that it is expensive and time consuming because the injections are performed multiple times per week. In addition, unlike some of the newer local injectable immunotherapy-type agents, intralesional IL-2 does not have a known systemic immune response (ie, bystander uninjected lesions typically do not regress). However, IL-2 remains a treatment option for patients with recurrent melanoma or in-transit disease.

PV-10/Rose Bengal

Rose bengal is a water-soluble xanthene dye that has long been used in liver function studies and to evaluate for ocular cell damage. PV-10 is a 10% solution of rose bengal that has been developed as an intralesional therapy for melanoma. Initial animal model studies have shown a response in tumors that have been injected as well as a bystander effect in those tumors that have not been directly injected.[34] These results have been corroborated by phase I and phase II trials. After promising results in the phase I trial of 11 patients showing an OR of 48% for injected lesions and 27% OR in bystander lesions, a phase II trial was undertaken.[35,36] In the phase II trial of 80 patients, an OR of 51% was seen, with a 26% CR and 25% PR. PV-10 has several potential advantages compared with other locoregional therapies, including prolonged long-term regression and a favorable toxicity profile.[36] Thirty-three percent of 21 subjects with evaluable bystander lesions achieved CR in these lesions, along with 10% PR and 14% stable disease, indicating a possible systemic immune response after PV-10 intralesional injection.[37] In the phase I study, only minor local skin and soft tissue adverse effects were reported.[35] In the phase II study, the first 40 patients treated had minimal side effects with only transient pain, vesicles, or edema and no grade 4 or 5 adverse events were reported.[38] When the final analysis was complete, 40% of patients had developed skin blistering, but this resolved in less than a month without sequelae.[36] Phase III studies are being planned as of April 2014.

Talimogene Laherparepvec

Talimogene laherparepvec (T-VEC) is an oncolytic herpes simplex virus encoded with the gene for GM-CSF. T-VEC is an injectable agent that has been studied in both a phase II and a phase III clinical trial in patients with stage III or IV metastatic melanoma. The phase II study showed an OR of 26% with a 16% CR and 10% PR. There was documented regression of the injected tumors as well as regression of bystander uninjected distant tumors. The tumor regression was maintained for 7 to 31 months in 92% of the responders.[39] The side effects were minimal, with the main adverse effect were transient flulike symptoms.[39] Results of the randomized phase III study of intralesional T-VEC or subcutaneous/systemic GM-CSF were presented at the American Society of Clinical Oncology meeting in 2013.[40] The results of the phase III study show that patients with metastatic disease who received intralesional T-VEC injections had an improved response compared with patients who received subcutaneous GM-CSF alone. Patients receiving T-VEC had an OR of 26.4% (95% confidence interval [CI] 21.4, 31.5) and a CR of 10.8% compared with an OR of 5.7% (95% CI 1.9, 9.5) and a CR of 0.7% for those treated with subcutaneous GM-CSF.[40] The durable response rate, meaning a PR or CR achieved for greater than 6 months, was 16.3% for patients treated with T-VEC and only 2.1% for patients treated with GM-CSF alone ($P<.0001$).[40] In addition, there was an improvement in median overall survival by 4.3 months, 23.3 months for T-VEC versus 19.0 months for GM-CSF (hazard ratio 0.79; 95% CI 0.61, 1.02; $P = .07$).[40] An interim planned analysis (released April 2014) of overall survival in 290 events in the phase III trial showed a further trend toward significance ($P = .051$). This trend toward an overall survival benefit suggests that, once the entire cohort of 430 patients (or all recorded events) is available for analysis, overall survival might become significant. Systemic bystander effects were seen in 34% of noninjected, nonvisceral metastases and 15% of noninjected visceral metastases, indicating that injection of T-VEC might produce some systemic immune response.[41] The adverse events associated with T-VEC are mild and were reported as only fatigue, chills, or pyrexia with no grade 3 adverse events occurring in more than 3% of the patients in either cohort (T-VEC vs GM-CSF alone).[40]

TOPICAL AGENTS

Imiquimod and diphencyprone cream (DPCP) are topically applied immunomodulators that have been investigated for the treatment of melanoma. Imiquimod is a toll-like receptor (TLR) agonist that activates TLR7 and induces cytokine secretion, which leads to downstream activation of effector cell and Th1 lymphocytes. The US Food and Drug Administration has approved its use for treatment of genital warts, actinic keratoses, and superficial basal cell carcinoma. Its use in the treatment of melanoma in-situ and metastatic melanoma has been documented in small case series and open-label studies.[42] In two small series, topical application of imiquimod with or without additional agents such as topical 5-fluorouracil, resulted in tumor regression rates of up to 90% for superficial lesions (**Table 3**).[43,44]

DPCP is a contact sensitizer that induces contact hypersensitivity and has been used to treat cutaneous warts and alopecia areata. The use of DPCP as a topical treatment of melanoma dates back to 1989. Its method of action in melanoma is not completely understood but it is thought that DPCP works via immunomodulation and activation of the thymus-derived TH17 lymphocytes. One of the largest series has recently been reported by Damian and colleagues.[45] This series included 50 patients with locally recurrent, in-transit, or dermal metastatic melanoma. Most patients had superficial dermal or epidermal disease and 40% had bulky cutaneous and subcutaneous disease. In the total cohort of 50 patients, 23 (46%) patients achieved a CR and an additional 19 (38%) patients showed a PR. Only 9 patients (18%) did not show any response. Recurrences developed in 6 of the patients with CR but this was treated with more intensive DPCP application. Patients with superficial dermal or epidermal disease had a better response: 61% showed a CR compared with only 21% of patients with bulky disease. The side effect profile of DPCP is tolerable, with skin reactions such as blistering and irritation being the most common side effect.

SYSTEMIC THERAPY

Systemic therapy may be an option for patients with progressive or unresponsive disease to previous locoregional therapies or even as a first-line therapy. The choice between starting with a regional approach such as perfusion-based or intralesion-based therapies versus a systemic approach revolves around a multidisciplinary discussion taking into account the individualization of the patient and disease characteristics. It is not a one-size-fits-all algorithm. Clinicians must take into account the numerous patient, disease/tumor and molecular analysis factors, as well as previous treatments, all of which play a role in helping to determine which initial or subsequent therapy is best. Recent advances in the systemic treatment of melanoma, such as the development of drugs that are classified as BRAF inhibitors (vemurafenib and dabrafenib), MEK inhibitors (trametinib), as well as systemic immunotherapy agents such as ipilimumab, have revolutionized the systemic therapy armamentarium for patients with metastatic melanoma.

RADIATION THERAPY

Melanoma has traditionally been considered to be radiation resistant to some extent, and current NCCN recommendations for the use of radiation therapy in the treatment

Table 3
Summary of response of common intralesional and topical treatment methods

Author, Year	Agent	Number Treated (N)	Response Rates (%)	Location of Response	Toxicity/Adverse Events (CTCAE Grade if Described in Publication)
Morton et al,[30] 1974	BCG	N = 45	OR: NR CR: 91 PR: NR	+ Tumor + Bystander	Fever, chills, localized abscess, lymphadenitis, systemic infection
Radny et al,[32] 2003	IL-2	N = 24	OR: 83.5 CR: 62.5 PR: 21	+ Tumor − Bystander	Grade 1: 69 events Grade 2: 31 events Grade 3: 1 event Grade 4: 0
Thompson et al,[35] 2008	PV-10	N = 11	OR: 48 CR: 36 PR: 12	+ Tumor + Bystander	Local skin reaction: mild pain, local inflammation, pruritus; 1 systemic AE (insomnia)
Agarwala et al,[36] 2013	PV-10	N = 80	OR: 51 CR: 26 PR: 25	+ Tumor + Bystander	Locoregional blistering 40%
Senzer et al,[39] 2009	T-VEC	N = 50	OR: 26 CR: 16 PR: 10	+ Tumor + Bystander	Grade 1 or 2: 85% Grade 3: 45 events Grade 4: 0 events
Andtbacka et al,[40] 2013	T-VEC	Stage IIIB/C, IV N = 436 N = 295 T-VEC N = 141 GM-CSF	T-VEC alone OR: 26.4 CR: 10.7 PR: 15.7	+ Tumor + Bystander	Fatigue, chills, pyrexia 26% serious AE <3% grade ≥3 AE
Florin et al,[44] 2012	Imiquimod	N = 5 45 Lesions	OR: 98 CR: 42 PR: 56	NR	NR
Damian et al,[45] 2014	Diphencyprone cream	N = 50 31 Thin/dermal 19 Bulky	OR: 84 CR: 46 PR: 38	+ Tumor + Lymph node and distant metastases	Local skin reaction: skin blistering, erythema

Abbreviations: AE, adverse event; BCG, Bacille Calmette-Guerin; CTCAE, Common Terminology Criteria for Adverse Events; GM-CSF, granulocyte macrophage-colony stimulating factor; NR, not reported.

of melanoma are limited to recurrent regional disease or as a palliative measure for unresectable nodal, in-transit, or satellite lesions. In patients with in-transit or regional recurrence, radiation may offer a significant benefit. Early studies evaluating outcomes after palliative radiation showed response rates of 60% to 70% for stage III disease.[46,47] Although a CR rate has been reported in only a small fraction of patients treated with radiation, and radiation does not prevent the development of distant metastatic disease, some studies have shown a significantly longer disease-free survival and overall survival in those patients who received radiation.[48,49] Treatment protocols are not well defined but the potential for symptom control makes radiation a viable option for patients with unresectable locoregional melanoma.

SUMMARY

Locoregional recurrence of melanoma is a complex problem that requires a multidisciplinary approach to management. If complete resection of all disease is possible, it is considered the standard of care and should be attempted. However, the burden of disease and the ability to render a patient NED are among the main determinants of treatment strategy. Several regionally directed treatment options exist that have been proven to achieve a CR in a high percentage of cases. Approaches can be intra-arterial perfusions such as ILI or HILP, which carry the highest OR (>80%) but obviously can only be used with in transit disease that is distal to the planned placement of the tourniquet on the extremity. Intralesional therapies such as PV-10 and T-VEC have the added advantage of treating dermal, subcutaneous, nodal, and even stage IV distant disease and can be applied to lesions that are injectable anywhere in the body, even performed under ultrasound or CT guidance. These compounds also have been shown to elicit a systemic immune response with documented distant bystander lesion responses in certain cases. The newer systemic agents have proved to be powerful, with rapid responses seen with BRAF and MEK inhibition and long-lasting durable responses seen with immunotherapy (ipilimumab). The ideal approach to these patients is likely to be combination therapy with local injectables or perfusional methods combined with a systemic approach to get a potential additive or synergistic effect for this complex and challenging clinical scenario.

Treatment must be individualized and take into consideration the extent of disease, tumor characteristics, and patient characteristics including age, comorbidities, previous therapies, and site of recurrence. Surgery, regional perfusions and intralesional injections all play a role in management options. These patients should be discussed and managed by a multidisciplinary team whenever possible.

REFERENCES

1. National Comprehensive Cancer Network. Melanoma. Version 3.2014. Available at: www.nccn.org. Accessed July 30, 2014.
2. Balch CM, Gershenwald JE, Soong S, et al. Final version of 2009 AJCC melanoma staging and classification. J Clin Oncol 2009;27:6199–206.
3. Pawlik TM, Ross MI, Johnson MM, et al. Predictors and natural history of in-transit melanoma after sentinel lymphadenectomy. Ann Surg Oncol 2005;12:587–96.
4. Coit DG, Andtbacka R, Anker CJ, et al. Melanoma. J Natl Compr Canc Netw 2012;10:366–400.
5. Squires MH 3rd, Delman KA. Current treatment of locoregional recurrence of melanoma. Curr Oncol Rep 2013;15:465–72.
6. Dong XD, Tyler D, Johnson JL, et al. Analysis of prognosis and disease progression after local recurrence of melanoma. Cancer 2000;88:1063–71.

7. Yao KA, Hsueh EC, Essner R, et al. Is sentinel lymph node mapping indicated for isolated local and in-transit recurrent melanoma? Ann Surg 2003;238: 743–7.

8. Beasley GM, Speicher P, Sharma K, et al. Efficacy of repeat sentinel lymph node biopsy in patients who develop recurrent melanoma. J Am Coll Surg 2014;21: 1435–40.

9. Creech O Jr, Krementz ET, Ryan RF, et al. Chemotherapy of cancer: regional perfusion utilizing an extracorporeal circuit. Ann Surg 1958;148:616–32.

10. Fraker DL. Management of in-transit melanoma of the extremity with isolated limb perfusion. Curr Treat Options Oncol 2004;5:173–84.

11. Fraker DL. Hyperthermic regional perfusion for melanoma and sarcoma of the limbs. Curr Probl Surg 1999;36:841–907.

12. Noorda EM, Vrouenraets BC, Nieweg OE, et al. Isolated limb perfusion for unresectable melanoma of the extremities. Arch Surg 2004;139:1237–42.

13. Kroon BB, Noorda EM, Vrouenraets BC, et al. Isolated limb perfusion for melanoma. J Surg Oncol 2002;79:252–5.

14. Eggermont AM, Schraffordt Koops H, Klausner JM, et al. Isolated limb perfusion with tumor necrosis factor and melphalan for limb salvage in 186 patients with locally advanced soft tissue extremity sarcomas. The cumulative multicenter European experience. Ann Surg 1996;224:756–64 [discussion: 764–5].

15. Cornett WR, McCall LM, Petersen RP, et al. Randomized multicenter trial of hyperthermic isolated limb perfusion with melphalan alone compared with melphalan plus tumor necrosis factor: American College of Surgeons Oncology Group Trial Z0020. J Clin Oncol 2006;24:4196–201.

16. Lienard D, Eggermont AM, Schraffordt Koops H, et al. Isolated perfusion of the limb with high-dose tumour necrosis factor-alpha (TNF-alpha), interferon-gamma (IFN-gamma) and melphalan for melanoma stage III. Results of a multi-centre pilot study. Melanoma Res 1994;4(Suppl 1):21–6.

17. Fraker DL, Alexander HR, Andrich M, et al. Treatment of patients with melanoma of the extremity using hyperthermic isolated limb perfusion with melphalan, tumor necrosis factor, and interferon gamma: results of a tumor necrosis factor dose-escalation study. J Clin Oncol 1996;14:479–89.

18. Moller MG, Lewis JM, Dessureault S, et al. Toxicities associated with hyperthermic isolated limb perfusion and isolated limb infusion in the treatment of melanoma and sarcoma. Int J Hyperthermia 2008;24:275–89.

19. Weiberdink J, Benckhuvsen C, Braat RP, et al. Dosimetry in isolation perfusion of the limbs by assessment of perfused tissue volume and grading of toxic tissue reactions. Eur J Cancer Clin Oncol 1982;18:905–10.

20. Eggimann P, Chiolero R, Chassot PG, et al. Systemic and hemodynamic effects of recombinant tumor necrosis factor alpha in isolation perfusion of the limbs. Chest 1995;107:1074–82.

21. Sorkin P, Abu-Abid S, Lev D, et al. Systemic leakage and side effects of tumor necrosis factor alpha administered via isolated limb perfusion can be manipulated by flow rate adjustment. Arch Surg 1995;130:1079–84.

22. Beasley GM, Petersen RP, Yoo J, et al. Isolated limb infusion for in-transit malignant melanoma of the extremity: a well-tolerated but less effective alternative to hyperthermic isolated limb perfusion. Ann Surg Oncol 2008;15:2195–205.

23. Raymond AK, Beasley GM, Broadwater G, et al. Current trends in regional therapy for melanoma: lessons learned from 225 regional chemotherapy treatments between 1995 and 2010 at a single institution. J Am Coll Surg 2011;213: 306–16.

24. Kroon HM, Moncrieff M, Kam PC, et al. Outcomes following isolated limb infusion for melanoma. A 14-year experience. Ann Surg Oncol 2008;15:3003–13.

25. Thompson JF, Kam PC, Waugh RC, et al. Isolated limb infusion with cytotoxic agents: a simple alternative to isolated limb perfusion. Semin Surg Oncol 1998;14:238–47.

26. Beasley GM, Caudle A, Petersen RP, et al. A multi-institutional experience of isolated limb infusion: defining response and toxicity in the US. J Am Coll Surg 2009;208:706–15 [discussion: 715–7].

27. Santillan AA, Delman KA, Beasley GM, et al. Predictive factors of regional toxicity and serum creatine phosphokinase levels after isolated limb infusion for melanoma: a multi-institutional analysis. Ann Surg Oncol 2009;16:2570–8.

28. Chai CY, Deneve JL, Beasley GM, et al. A multi-institutional experience of repeat regional chemotherapy for recurrent melanoma of extremities. Ann Surg Oncol 2012;19:1637–43.

29. Kroon HM, Lin DY, Kam PC, et al. Efficacy of repeat isolated limb infusion with melphalan and actinomycin D for recurrent melanoma. Cancer 2009;115: 1932–40.

30. Morton DL, Eilber FR, Holmes EC, et al. BCG immunotherapy of malignant melanoma: summary of a seven-year experience. Ann Surg 1974;180:635–43.

31. Agarwala SS, Neuberg D, Park Y, et al. Mature results of a phase III randomized trial of bacillus Calmette-Guerin (BCG) versus observation and BCG plus dacarbazine versus BCG in the adjuvant therapy of American Joint Committee on Cancer Stage I-III melanoma (E1673): a trial of the Eastern Oncology Group. Cancer 2004;100:1692–8.

32. Radny P, Caroli JM, Bauer J, et al. Phase II trial of intralesional therapy with interleukin-2 in soft-tissue melanoma metastases. Br J Cancer 2003;89: 1620–6.

33. Elias EG, Sharma BK. Consequential administration of intralesional (intratumoral) GM-CSF and IL-2 in the management of metastatic and primary invasive cutaneous melanoma. J Clin Oncol 2013;(Suppl) [abstract: e20052].

34. Toomey P, Kodumudi K, Weber A, et al. Intralesional injection of rose bengal induces a systemic tumor-specific immune response in murine models of melanoma and breast cancer. PLoS One 2013;8:e68561.

35. Thompson JF, Hersey P, Wachter E. Chemoablation of metastatic melanoma using intralesional rose Bengal. Melanoma Res 2008;18:405–11.

36. Agarwala SS, Thompson JF, Smithers BM, et al. Locoregional disease control in metastatic melanoma: exploratory analysis from phase 2 testing of intralesional rose Bengal. ECCO-ESMO-ESTRO Congress. Amsterdam, September 2013 [abstract: 3755].

37. Agarwala SS, Thompson JF, Smithers BM, et al. Chemoablation of metastatic melanoma with rose bengal (PV-10). J Clin Oncol 2010;28(Suppl):15s [abstract: 8534].

38. Agarwala SS, Thompson JF, Smithers BM, et al. Chemoablation of melanoma with intralesional rose Bengal (PV-10). J Clin Oncol 2009;(Suppl) [abstract: 9060].

39. Senzer NN, Kaufman HL, Amatruda T, et al. Phase II clinical trial of a granulocyte-macrophage colony-stimulating factor-encoding, second-generation oncolytic herpesvirus in patients with unresectable metastatic melanoma. J Clin Oncol 2009;27:5763–71.

40. Andtbacka RH, Collichio FA, Amatruda T, et al. OPTiM: a randomized phase 3 trial of talimogene laherparepvec (T-VEC) vs subcutaneous (SC) granulocyte-macrophage colony-stimulating factor (GM-CSF) for the treatment (tx) of

unresected stage IIIB/C and IV melanoma. J Clin Oncol 2013;31(Suppl) [abstract: LBA9008].

41. Andtbacka RH, Ross MI, Delman K, et al. Responses of injected and uninjected lesions to intralesional talimogene laherparepvec (T-VEC) in the OPTiM study and the contribution of surgery to response. Society of Surgical Oncology Annual Meeting. Phoenix, March 2014.

42. Ellis LZ, Cohen JL, High W, et al. Melanoma in situ treated successfully using imiquimod after nonclearance with surgery: review of the literature. Dermatol Surg 2012;38:937–46.

43. Berman B, Poochareon VN, Villa AM. Novel dermatologic uses of the immune response modifier imiquimod 5% cream. Skin Therapy Lett 2002;7:1–6.

44. Florin V, Desmedt E, Vercambre-Darras S, et al. Topical treatment of cutaneous metastases of malignant melanoma using combined imiquimod and 5-fluorouracil. Invest New Drugs 2012;30:1641–5.

45. Damian DL, Saw RP, Thompson JF. Topical immunotherapy with diphencyprone for in transit and cutaneously metastatic melanoma. J Surg Oncol 2014;109: 308–13.

46. Sause WT, Cooper JS, Rush S, et al. Fraction size in external beam radiation therapy in the treatment of melanoma. Int J Radiat Oncol Biol Phys 1991;20: 429–32.

47. Seegenschmiedt MH, Keilholz L, Altendorf-Hofmann A, et al. Palliative radiotherapy for recurrent and metastatic malignant melanoma: prognostic factors for tumor response and long-term outcome: a 20-year experience. Int J Radiat Oncol Biol Phys 1999;44:607–18.

48. Olivier KR, Schild SE, Morris CG, et al. A higher radiotherapy dose is associated with more durable palliation and longer survival in patients with metastatic melanoma. Cancer 2007;110:1791–5.

49. Konefal JB, Emami B, Pilepich MV. Malignant melanoma: analysis of dose fractionation in radiation therapy. Radiology 1987;164:607–10.

50. Coventry BJ, Kroon HM, Giles MH, et al. Australian multi-center experience outside of the Sydney Melanoma Unit of isolated limb infusion chemotherapy for melanoma. J Surg Oncol 2014;109(8):780–5. http://dx.doi.org/10.1002/jso.23590.

51. Wong J, Chen YA, Fisher KJ, et al. Isolated limb infusion in a series of over 100 infusions: a single-center experience. Ann Surg Oncol 2013;20(4):1121–7. http://dx.doi.org/10.1245/s10434-012-2782-8.

Melanoma Vaccines
Mixed Past, Promising Future

Junko Ozao-Choy, MD, Delphine J. Lee, MD, PhD, Mark B. Faries, MD*

KEYWORDS

- Melanoma • Vaccine • Immunomodulator • Adjuvant • Immunotherapy

KEY POINTS

- Numerous vaccine antigen sources have been evaluated, and each has advantages and disadvantages.
- Most phase 3 vaccine trials have not shown clinical benefit, although there have been a few successes and suggestions of activity.
- Novel vaccine strategies using the tumor in vivo as an antigen source bypass the need to define tumor antigens; allow simple, yet personalized therapy; and are perhaps the most interesting current method of vaccination.
- Numerous immunomodulators are now available or in development that could enhance vaccination.
- Adequate immune monitoring with clinically meaningful surrogate end points are critical for additional vaccine development.

INTRODUCTION

Vaccination is the earliest form of immunotherapy, corresponding to the discovery of the immune system itself, and infectious disease vaccinations are perhaps the greatest advance in the history of medicine. Vaccination for cancer has been more difficult, although it had auspicious and early beginnings. The first attempt predates our knowledge of the specific mechanisms involved in vaccination. In the late nineteenth century, William B. Coley, a surgeon in New York at the time, was deeply saddened by the death of a 17-year-old patient with metastatic Ewing sarcoma, spurring him to

Supported in part by fellowship funding from the Patricia Brown Foundation (Dr Ozao-Choy), and by funding from John Wayne Cancer Institute Auxiliary (Santa Monica, CA), Dr Miriam & Sheldon G. Adelson Medical Research Foundation (Boston, MA), The Borstein Family Foundation (Los Angeles, CA) and National Cancer Institute grant P01 CA29605. The content is solely the responsibility of the authors and does not necessarily represent the official view of the National Cancer Institute or the National Institutes of Health.
John Wayne Cancer Institute, 2200 Santa Monica Boulevard, Santa Monica, CA 90404, USA
* Corresponding author.
E-mail address: mark.faries@jwci.org

Surg Clin N Am 94 (2014) 1017–1030
http://dx.doi.org/10.1016/j.suc.2014.07.005
0039-6109/14/$ – see front matter © 2014 Elsevier Inc. All rights reserved.

surgical.theclinics.com

begin to look for novel therapies to treat cancer.[1,2] He was struck by the case of a patient who had tumor regression after developing erysipelas.[3] He wondered if this phenomenon was caused by the infection and then took it on himself to begin inoculating patients with streptococcal organisms in 1891. He reported tumor regression in numerous patients. Coley continued to refine his therapy by using a heat-killed *Streptococcus* and *Serratia* combination, which became known as Coley toxin.[1] This administration of an immune adjuvant to the site of a superficial tumor is perhaps the first example of cancer vaccination, albeit using the existing tumor as antigen source. This strategy has interesting echoes in melanoma immunotherapy, as is discussed later.

More than a century later, Coley's vision of therapeutic immunology is a reality, with the approval of several immune agents in melanoma, and additional promising therapies moving through the development pipeline. However, vaccines continue to present difficulties, showing consistent benefit. Although several negative vaccine trials have led many to discount the possibility of effective cancer vaccination, there are hopeful signs that continued research efforts are not only justified but important components of the overall effort to develop effective therapies for melanoma and other cancers. After several decades of failed attempts at developing potent therapeutic vaccines, the first proof-of-concept cancer vaccine Sipeucel-T was approved for use in patients who have prostate cancer by the US Food and Drug Administration in 2010,[4,5] and as discussed later, a trial of peptide vaccination in melanoma[6] showed a significant survival advantage in the vaccine group.

Increased knowledge of the immune system and its interaction with tumors, along with a widening array of clinically available immunomodulators, make the prospect of effective vaccines increasingly likely. Over several decades, breakthroughs in basic science and an increased knowledge about the role of antibodies in infection have made many surmise that vaccination and the establishment of antitumor antibodies may be a possible strategy to cure cancer.[7] Many cancers have been studied extensively with respect to vaccine treatment but, perhaps, no cancer as extensively as melanoma.

Vaccine strategies are highly varied and may be characterized by the antigen source and the adjuvants or immune modulators given with the antigen. Much of the early period of vaccine development was characterized by substantial debate regarding the ideal antigen. Options vary from the simplest peptide vaccines to the most complex autologous whole-tumor cells. Each approach has advantages and disadvantages (**Fig. 1, Table 1**). Generally, simple peptide vaccines are easier to prepare, store, administer, and monitor, but they offer the narrowest spectrum of tumor targets and are potentially relevant to fewer patients. More complex vaccines are the most likely to offer antigens that are relevant to any given patient, but are more difficult to produce and administer. They also present substantial difficulties in monitoring immune responses, because those responses may be varied among different individuals. It is becoming increasingly apparent that the nature of the antigen is only a part of the story, perhaps a small part. What may be more significant is the context of the immune stimulation in terms of both patient characteristics and immunologic adjuvants or other immunomodulators. Modification of these factors could prove more important than the specific source of antigen for a vaccine.

Autologous Melanoma Vaccines

In autologous vaccines, the patient's own tumor is used as the antigen source. There are several significant advantages to autologous vaccines. First, because the source of antigen is the patient's own tumor, there is, by definition, an HLA-type match,

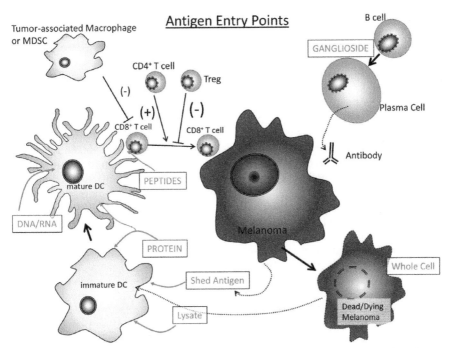

Fig. 1. Antigen entry points: numerous options exist for vaccine antigen, and each may enter at a different point in immune response development. Peptides, the simplest antigen, enter at the immunologic synapse between T-cell and antigen-presenting cell and do not require processing. Others require uptake, processing, and presentation to be recognized. Antigen may also be released from dead or dying cancer cells, either injected as a prepared vaccine or produced from existing metastases. MDSC, myeloid-derived suppressor cells.

ensuring that antigen presentation is adequate. Second, the vaccines are likely to contain antigens that are unique to that particular patient and, thus, are personalized. However, the derivation of vaccine from an autologous source is daunting from a practical standpoint, and there is little consensus about the optimal method. In addition,

Table 1
Antigen types

Antigen Type	Pros	Cons
Peptide	Easy preparation Easy storage Simple monitoring	Narrow antigen spectrum HLA restriction Many limited to class I presentation
Protein	No HLA restriction Simple preparation	Requires antigen cross-presentation to sensitize CD8 T cells Still fairly narrow antigen spectrum
DNA/RNA	Simple preparation No HLA restriction	May be difficult to generate both CD4 and CD8 responses Requires delivery of genetic material

Ganglioside	Immune monitoring (antibody
	  response) is simple
		Relies largely on humeral response
		  for effect

Lysate	Broad antigen spectrum	Preparation/storage more difficult
Whole cell	Most diverse antigen spectrum	Preparation/storage most difficult

sufficient tumor must be available to provide raw material for the vaccine. Thus, patients who have low tumor burden or those who have undergone complete resection of their disease are not candidates for this type of therapy. Melanoma metastases may be genetically and antigenically heterogeneous within any given patient.[8] This factor could create a situation in which a single metastasis, used for vaccine preparation, would not contain enough antigenic diversity to lead to a protective response against every metastatic focus.

An early autologous vaccine to undergo phase 3 trial was of a heat shock protein gp96 peptide complex (HSPPC-96) vaccine derived from autologous tumor.[9,10] Heat shock proteins are soluble, intracellular sticky proteins and bind peptides, including antigenic peptides generated within cells. They are believed to play an important role as chaperones for antigen presentation, required for instructing the antigen-specific antitumor immune responses. When heat shock proteins are purified from tumors, noncovalent complexes of these proteins along with peptides expressed by the tumor cell are obtained. When injected into the skin, heat shock proteins may interact with antigen-presenting cells through CD91, a heat shock protein receptor. This process leads to re-presentation of heat shock protein–chaperoned peptides by major histocompatibility complex (MHC) proteins as well as stimulation and maturation of antigen-presenting cells. Despite their extracellular location on administration, the tumor-associated peptides bound to gp96 may gain access to presentation on MHC class I (cross-priming), important for activation of antitumor killer T-cell responses.

The phase 3 trial[10] studied in 322 patients at 71 centers and randomly assigned patients 2:1 to receive either the vaccine or physician choice of dacarbazine, temozolomide, interleukin 2 (IL-2), or complete tumor resection. There was no difference in overall survival (OS), although patients with M1a or M1b disease who received more than 10 doses of vaccine survived longer than those receiving fewer treatments. Although this type of analysis may be biased, the investigators attempted to control for such bias using landmark analysis. In addition, preclinical models suggested that at least 4 doses of the vaccine would be required to stimulate a protective immune response. The investigators concluded that this M1a and M1b subset of patients may be candidates for further study, and this vaccination strategy remains an area of interest.[11] However, there is also a theoretic concern that chronic stimulation with antigen may lead to tolerance, rather than effective immunity, and the ideal duration of cancer vaccination in patients remains unclear. Other whole-cell autologous vaccines include those developed by Berd and colleagues,[12] subsequently evaluated in clinical trials as M-Vax. This vaccine uses the patient's irradiated melanoma cells, which are modified with dinitrophenyl, a hapten, which previous research suggests helps improve antigen visibility.[13] The treatment program consists of multiple intradermal injections of 2,4-dinitrophenol (DNP)-modified autologous tumor cells mixed with bacille Calmette-Guérin (BCG) as an immunologic adjuvant. Administration of DNP vaccine to patients with metastatic melanoma induces the development of inflammation in metastases.[14] In a phase 3 trial, which has completed accrual, patients were assigned to M-Vax or placebo followed by low-dose IL-2. Primary end points were best overall tumor response and survival at 2 years. The trial was suspended in 2009, and results have yet to be published. Another autologous, whole-cell strategy was developed by Dillman and colleagues[15] and consists of resected tumor cells, which are cultured in vitro and irradiated before administration. This vaccine has not been evaluated in phase 3 studies (**Table 2**).

An alternative to whole-cell autologous vaccines is the use of tumor lysates pulsed onto dendritic cells (DCs). DCs are specialized leukocytes, which are the most potent generators of de novo antigen-specific immune responses. Although several immune cells are capable of presenting antigens to activate effector cells, the use of DCs as an

Table 2
Phase 3 trials of melanoma vaccines

Author, Year	n	Arms	Hazard Ratio	Confidence Interval	P Value	Notes
Kirkwood et al,[25] 2001	880	High-dose interferon vs GM-2KLH/QS-21	RFS: 1.47 OS: 1.52	(1.14–1.90) (1.07–2.15)	.0015 .009	
Hersey et al,[17] 2002	700	Vaccinia melanoma cell lysate vs observation	RFS: 0.86 OS: 0.81	(0.7–1.07) (0.64–1.02)	.17 .068	
Sondak et al,[19] 2002	698	Melacine vs observation	0.84 (recurrence or death)	(0.66–1.08)	.17	HLA-A2+, C3+ significant
Schadendorf et al,[36] 2004	108	DC+ peptides vs dacarbacine	OS		.48	AWD stage IV
Morton et al,[22] 2007	1160	Canvaxin vs placebo	1.26		.040	Stage III
Morton et al,[22] 2007	496	Canvaxin vs placebo	1.29	(0.97–1.72)	.086	Stage IV
Testori et al,[10] 2008	322	Hsp96 vaccine vs BAC			.316	Stage IV
Hodi et al,[29] 2010	676	Ipilimumab vs peptide vs both	OS: 1.04		.76	AWD
Lawson et al,[30] 2010	398	GM-CSF ± peptides	OS: 0.94 DFS: 0.93	(0.70–1.26) (0.73–1.27)	.670 .709	
Schwartzentruber et al,[6] 2011	185	IL-2 ± peptides	RR PFS OS		.03 .008 .06	AWD, all favor vaccine
Eggermont et al,[26] 2013	1314	GM2-KLH/QS-21 vs observation	RFS: 1.03 OS: 1.66	(0.84–1.25) (0.90–1.51)	.81 .25	
Suriano et al,[18] 2013	250	Vaccinia melanoma oncolysate vs vaccinia	OS		.70	
Unpublished data, 2013	?	MAGE-A3 vs placebo	OS		NS	Subgroups pending

Abbreviations: AWD, alive with disease; BAC, best alternative care; DC, dendritic cells; DFS, disease-free survival; KLH-QS-21, keyhole limpet hemocyanin and the QS-21 adjuvant; NS, not significant; PFS, progression-free survival; RFS, recurrence-free survival; RR, relative risk.

immune adjuvant for tumor vaccination may provide a more potent source of immune activation. A randomized phase 2 comparison of autologous tumor antigen-pulsed DCs versus autologous whole-cell vaccination showed a survival advantage in the DC arm (hazard ratio [HR], 0.27; 95% confidence interval [CI], 0.098–0.729).[16] Additional considerations of DC vaccines are considered later.

Allogeneic Vaccines

The use of vaccines derived from stock melanoma cell lines has several theoretic advantages over autologous vaccines. First, the vaccine may be prepared before a patient's need for treatment, eliminating the delay in therapy required when deriving cells from resected tumors. Second, the cells used in the vaccine can be preselected for high antigen expression. Third, the presence of foreign alloantigens could stimulate a more potent immune response than that engendered by autologous tumor. Several allogeneic whole-cell or whole-cell lysate vaccines have been evaluated in phase 3 clinical trials, including those using vaccinia melanoma cell lysate (VMCL), vaccinia melanoma oncolysate (VMO), Melacine, and Canvaxin.

The VMCL vaccine uses a single melanoma cell line, which is lysed in vitro using vaccinia virus and injected intradermally. Infection of melanoma cells with vaccinia virus could provide additional stimulation of antitumor immunity by introducing viral pattern recognition ligands in the vaccine. The phase 3 trial[17] included 700 patients in Australia and was randomized 1:1 against observation as control. Data were analyzed with a median of 8 years of follow-up and showed a nonsignificantly increased OS in the vaccine group (5-year OS, 60.6% vaccine vs 54.8% control; HR, 0.81; 95% CI, 0.64–1.02, $P = .068$). The patients in the control arm also showed longer survival compared with that expected for the time, a seemingly common phenomenon in melanoma vaccine trials.

The next large trial of a whole-cell lysate was the VMO vaccine. This trial consisted of a lysate of 4 melanoma cell lines and 250 patients from 11 North American institutions, who were randomized to vaccine or vaccinia only. A study of the long-term results of the trial was published in 2013 and showed no indication of benefit (or harm) for the vaccine group.[18]

A third phase 3 trial[19] was conducted by the Southwest Oncology Group and evaluated Melacine, a lysate of 2 melanoma cell lines combined with a detoxified Freund adjuvant (DETOX). Freund adjuvant comprises mycobacterial components, which are potent immune stimulators. The study enrolled 689 patients, who were randomized to vaccine or to observation. The study showed an HR of 0.84 in favor of the vaccine arm, but the difference was not statistically significant. However, examination of subgroups with cross-reactivity with the HLA types presented in the vaccine, particularly HLA-A2-positive and HLA-C3-positive patients, showed a significant advantage.[20] If allogeneic tumor cells were to be used for further tumor vaccine development, perhaps some level of matching to the recipient's MHC could improve the efficacy of the vaccine. Melacine was approved for use in Canada for stage IV melanoma, based on improved quality of life compared with combination chemotherapy. It was not approved in the United States or elsewhere.

The largest phase 3 clinical experience for an allogeneic whole-cell vaccine is with Canvaxin.[21] Canvaxin consists of 3 melanoma cell lines, selected for their spectrum of antigen expression and irradiated at doses so that the cells would be live but replication incompetent on administration. The vaccine showed excellent results in phase 2 trials and was evaluated in 2 large, randomized trials in resected stage III and stage IV melanoma. Patients were randomized to vaccine or placebo, with both arms receiving BCG as an immune adjuvant with the first 2 doses. The trial in stage III patients enrolled 1160 patients, and the stage IV study enrolled 496.[22] Both trials were halted after interim analyses for futility, because there was no significant difference from placebo.

The Canvaxin studies reported outcomes in the vaccine arms that were similar to those predicted by phase 2 results.[23] These vaccine survival times, which were superior to historical controls and seemed better than those of other contemporary adjuvant therapy trials, were no better than those of the control group, who received only BCG. Although BCG had been evaluated as an immune adjuvant in melanoma before, previous trials used relatively ineffective administration schemes and were inadequately powered to evaluate the therapy. Survival times of the control arms of the study were longer than the vaccine arm, although these values were not technically statistically different at the threshold of an interim analysis (stage III $P = .040$, stage IV $P = .086$). It is possible that this vaccine strategy and others could be improved with optimization of dosing and schedule, because chronic, repeated inoculation with tumor antigens may lead to less robust antitumor responses and instead induce tolerance to tumor antigens. However, the OS of all patients both in the treated and control arms was longer than expected, indicating that participation in the protocol was not harmful.

Ganglioside Vaccines

Gangliosides are glycolipids that are differentially expressed in several cancer types. Thus, they are also potential targets as tumor-specific antigens for immune therapy or vaccination.[24] Two large phase 3 trials have been performed using the GM2 ganglioside. The first of these trials[25] was conducted by the Easter Cooperative Oncology Group in collaboration with the North American cooperative groups. This study compared GM2 vaccine (consisting of the ganglioside coupled to keyhole limpet hemocyanin [KLH] and the QS-21 adjuvant) with high-dose interferon-α2b. The trial enrolled 880 patients and reported superior relapse-free survival and OS in the interferon arm.

The second trial was performed by the European Organization for Research and Treatment of Cancer[26] and randomized patients to either GM2-KLH-QS21 vaccine or observation. The trial included 1314 patients and was halted at the second interim analysis for futility, because early follow-up showed no suggestion of a relapse-free survival advantage to the vaccine group and a possible OS disadvantage. With additional follow-up, the survival curves are almost overlapping, indicating that although there was no harm by vaccination, there was clearly no benefit.

Peptide Vaccines

Peptides are perhaps the most commonly used tumor-associated antigen source for melanoma vaccines. These protein fragments are normally presented in the context of MHC proteins to be recognized by T lymphocytes. Cancer-specific peptides were identified in melanoma more than 2 decades ago.[27,28] The peptides are easily produced, stored, and administered. Because of the narrow spectrum of immune responses possible to the peptides, immunologic monitoring of peptide vaccination is straightforward. In part because of these advantages, several dozen peptide vaccine trials have been performed in melanoma, including 3 randomized phase 3 trials.[6,29,30]

However, the simplicity of these antigens is also a potential weakness. Each peptide generally contains only 1 epitope for the immune system to target, and peptides are limited in compatibility to HLA-matched patients. Because HLA-A2 is a common allele in patients with melanoma, most peptide vaccine studies conducted have been limited to peptides that bind HLA-A2 and therefore have been available only to HLA-A2$^+$ patients. In addition, with a narrow spectrum of target epitopes, the potential for antigen loss through immune selection and survival of antigen-negative clones is a concern. With identification of numerous potential peptide antigens with histocompatibility for several HLA types, some of this limitation has been at least partially overcome.[31] It is still not clear whether those improvements will translate into increased effectiveness in the clinical setting. Despite the relative ease of peripheral blood monitoring of immunization, correlations of successful immunization by such monitoring and clinical outcomes have been limited or even inverse (ie, lower peripheral blood responses in clinical responders).[32,33] It is also possible that the in vitro assays used thus far to monitor peripheral blood responses lack the relevant immune readouts that correlate to clinical benefit.

The results of 3 phase 3 trials of peptide vaccination have been mixed. All 3 trials included a systemic immunomodulating drug and examined the effect of adding peptide vaccines. One[6] examined high-dose IL-2, an approved therapy for metastatic melanoma, with or without gp100 peptide and incomplete Freund adjuvant in patients with measurable metastatic disease. The multicenter trial enrolled 185 patients and reported a significant improvement in the overall response rate (16% vs 6%, $P = .03$) and progression-free survival (2.2 vs 1.6 months, $P = .008$) in the vaccine group. The trend in median OS was improved in the gp100 group compared with the IL-2 alone group, but was not statistically significant (17.8 vs 11.1 months, $P = .06$). Thus, this is the first peptide vaccine to show a clinical benefit in a phase 3 trial.

Another trial[30] examined the role of both a peptide vaccine and granulocyte-macrophage colony-stimulating factor (GM-CSF) as adjuvant therapies in patients with resected stage III and IV melanoma. This trial enrolled 815 patients, who were assigned to one of the multiple arms of the trial depending on their HLA-A2 status. Only HLA-A2+ patients (n = 398) were randomized to receive vaccine or peptide placebo. The study has been reported only in abstract form, and mature results are expected in 2014. Preliminary results reported a relapse-free survival advantage with GM-CSF, but this finding has lost statistical significance over time and was not accompanied by an OS benefit. The addition of peptide vaccination did not seem to improve OS or relapse-free survival.

The third phase 3 trial[29] involving peptide vaccination was conducted within a larger trial evaluating the efficacy of cytotoxic T-lymphocyte antigen 4 (CTLA-4) blockade with ipilimumab. The trial had 3 arms: gp100 peptide alone (n = 136), ipilimumab alone (n = 137), and the combination (n = 403). The trial showed a significant survival advantage to ipilimumab but no advantage to peptide vaccination. This study provides an interesting contrast to the trial of peptide vaccination in the context of IL-2, which did show a benefit, and highlights the paramount importance of context to determine the clinical impact of an immune therapy. The mixed results of these 3 peptide vaccine trials indicate that additional work is required to optimize vaccine strategies using peptides.

IMMUNE ADJUVANTS AND IMMUNOMODULATORS

Although this review has been focused on the types of antigen sources that have been used in melanoma vaccines; an equally important, if not more important, consideration may be the context of immunization with regard to the patient population, the frequency of dosing, and the immune adjuvant and immunomodulators that are given with the vaccine. As knowledge of the immune system and its interaction with melanoma has improved, new opportunities for rational immunization improvement have arisen (**Fig. 2**).

Vaccines, including many infectious disease vaccines, are given with nonspecific immune adjuvants to boost immunologic responses. Vaccine adjuvants serve to increase recognition of antigens, amplify immune responses, and modulate those responses. Many early trials used traditional vaccine adjuvants, such as incomplete Freund, whereas others used live or killed microorganism components such as BCG[21] or detoxified mycobacterial cell walls (eg, DETOX).[19] The discovery of toll-like receptors and elucidation of their importance in the development of immune responses has led to incorporation of their ligands into some vaccination strategies.

One of the most promising areas of enhancing vaccine responsiveness is the use of DCs as immune adjuvants.[34] These cells are primarily responsible for generation of new responses in vivo. DCs may be obtained from bone marrow, but for clinical trials

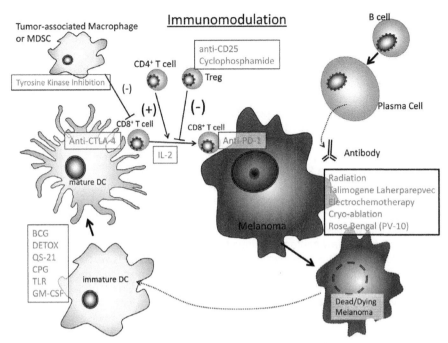

Fig. 2. Immunomodulation: the spectrum of available agents to boost or modify immune responses has increased dramatically in recent years and can interact with the system in numerous places.

are most commonly derived from peripheral blood mononuclear cells. Early studies of DC vaccines showed encouraging response rates in patients with relatively advanced melanoma. Nestle and colleagues[35] used autologous DCs cultured in GM-CSF and IL-4 and then pulsed with tumor lysates or peptides before infusion into 16 patients with advanced melanoma. Two of 16 patients had a complete response (CR), whereas 3 of 16 patients had a partial response (PR). More recently, a DC vaccine was evaluated in a phase 3 trial of 108 patients.[36] The DCs in this trial were pulsed with peptides, and the control arm was treated with dacarbazine chemotherapy. There was no indication of benefit to vaccination, and the trial was closed at the recommendation of the Data Safety Monitoring Board.

However, it has now become clear that not all DCs are the same. Depending on the state of maturation of the DCs, and the cytokines and chemokines they produce, the cells may not traffic well to present antigen and may skew immune responses toward tolerance. This new knowledge is being incorporated into the design of current DC vaccine trials in melanoma and other cancers.[37]

In a recent pilot trial, DCs were grown with GM-CSF, IL-4, tumor necrosis factor (TNF), and CD40 ligand (CD40L).[38] Both TNF and CD40L are important for maturation of DCs. The DCs were then pulsed with allogeneic, killed melanoma cells. Of 20 patients with advanced melanoma who were vaccinated, 1 showed a CR, whereas another had a PR. This study was proof of concept that HLA restriction could be overcome by loading mature DCs with allogeneic killed melanoma cells.

Additional DC vaccine trials are planned, including 2 upcoming phase 3 trials. There is hope that improved understanding of DC biology will increase the benefits of vaccination for these studies.

INTRALESIONAL IMMUNOTHERAPY: TUMOR (IN SITU) AS VACCINE

We have characterized Coley intralesional injection of bacterial toxins as vaccination, although the injection itself did not contain tumor antigens. Rather, the antigens were already present, and he simply added the adjuvant. A similar strategy was pursued by Morton and colleagues[39] starting in the 1960s using BCG. In the first such case, a woman presented with numerous in transit metastases on her upper extremity. Her other arm had been paralyzed by polio, and so she declined an amputation. Morton, who was in the early stages of developing an allogeneic whole-cell vaccine at the time, elected to inject BCG into her melanoma lesions, using the lesion as vaccine. Subsequently, all of her lesions, both injected and noninjected, regressed completely. She remained free of disease for many years thereafter.

BCG was explored with great enthusiasm after early publications of melanoma regression.[40] Subsequent reports documented regression of noninjected metastases, even at visceral sites.[41] However, severe toxicities, including disseminated intravascular coagulation, anaphylaxis, and death were reported, and enthusiasm for the technique waned.[42,43] A few centers continue to use BCG in this way, although at greatly reduced doses, and it is included in the National Comprehensive Cancer Network guidelines as an option for in transit disease.[44] A recent report used the combination of BCG and imiquimod, the topical toll-like receptor agonist, and reported regression of extensive areas of in transit metastases, with minimal toxicity.[45]

Although radiation is generally understood to be immunosuppressive, it may also have local immunostimulatory effects, such as increased antigen expression or release. Local radiation therapy may facilitate development of systemic immunity, something known as the abscopal effect. An example of this effect was recently reported in the context of a patient previously treated with ipilimumab.[46] Although it is difficult to rule out the possibility of a delayed clinical response to checkpoint blockade, numerous similar examples, and biologically promising mechanisms suggest that radiation may be a fruitful avenue for further study to stimulate antitumor immune responses. Several clinical trials are evaluating local therapies such as radiation or regional chemotherapy administration as adjuncts to systemic immunotherapies.

Another developing local immunotherapy is talimogene laherparepvec (T-VEC), an oncolytic herpes simplex virus, which was engineered to express GM-CSF.[47] Tumor destruction is believed to stem from both the oncolytic effect of the herpes simplex virus, which causes the melanoma cell to lyse, and GM-CSF, which is expressed on infection and may attract and activate DCs to present antigens from the tumor lysate, inducing an antitumor immune response.[47–49] Recently, the results of the OPTiM trial,[50] a phase 3 randomized control trial comparing T-VEC with GM-CSF alone, was presented at a meeting of the American Society of Clinical Oncology. Unresectable stage IIIB/C or stage IV patients with injectable cutaneous, subcutaneous, or nodal lesions were randomized to intralesional T-VEC or subcutaneous GM-CSF. The objective response rate (ORR) with T-VEC was 26%, with 11% CR, compared with GM-CSF alone, which had a 6% ORR and 1% CR. Durable response rate for T-VEC was 16% compared with 2% for GM-SCF. Interim OS analysis showed a trend in benefit toward T-VEC. Thus, T-VEC is the first such melanoma local immune therapy to show benefit in OS in a phase 3 randomized clinical trial in melanoma.

FUTURE

Although many of the clinical trials evaluating melanoma vaccines have not shown a benefit, and some have even raised concerns that vaccination can be harmful, there are many reasons to support that vaccines will be an important component of optimal therapy for melanoma in the future. Successful deployment of melanoma vaccines was probably hampered because they were the first immune therapies to be developed. Introduction in an era of less sophisticated knowledge of tumor immunology and clinical trial design led to studies conducted with insufficient sample sizes or in populations that could not be accurately stratified because of inadequate staging. Despite these challenges, some successes have kept cancer vaccination research alive. Hopeful signs include 2 positive randomized trials in the peptide/IL-2 study[6] and the T-VEC trial[49] as well as the availability of new and increasingly diverse immunomodulators.

Perhaps the most important challenge that faces vaccine development is the identification of reliable surrogates for clinical outcomes. Traditionally, clinical development begins with preclinical investigations, and many early phase trials use surrogates, such as immune end points, to select therapies to take forward. This model seems to be unreliable in melanoma vaccines. For example, preclinical models had suggested a strong synergy between peptide vaccination and checkpoint blockade with anti-CTLA-4 antibody but this theory was not borne out by the completed phase 3 trial. Numerous immune surrogates have been used to guide modification and combination of immune therapies. One example is that of GM-CSF, which leads to improved antibody responses, but not to improved clinical outcomes in multiple randomized trials.[51] Another is the measurement of number of circulating antigen-specific lymphocytes. In a study performed at the National Cancer Institute, several cytokines were added to peptide vaccines, and peripheral blood responses were monitored. The only group with significant clinical responses, that in which peptides were combined with IL-2, had decreased numbers of circulating antigen-specific cells.[32] Development of other measures of productive antitumor responses is needed and may include evaluation of tumor material to assess immune infiltrates or downregulation of immunosuppressive factors. The current wealth of agents that are potentially useful as adjuncts to vaccination are most welcome but will require improved means of assessment to sort through. Reliance on large randomized trials with survival end points will be too slow to provide answers in the time frame that many patients need.

Coley's vision of curing cancer through vaccination has become a reality for some patients.[4] The advent of new immune agents and new means of applying immunotherapies make the prospect of extending benefits to more patients increasingly likely. We should remember Coley's pioneering spirit, including the courage and tenacity that he needed to inject patients with his toxin, as we enter a critical second phase of melanoma vaccine development.

REFERENCES

1. Coley W. The treatment of malignant tumors by repeated inoculations of erysipelas: with a report of ten original cases. New York: Lea Brothers; 1893.
2. Coley W. Treatment of inoperable malignant tumors with the toxins of erysipelas and the bacillus prodigiosus. Trans Am Surg Assoc 1894;12:183.
3. McCarthy EF. The toxins of William B. Coley and the treatment of bone and soft-tissue sarcomas. Iowa Orthop J 2006;26:154–8.
4. Kantoff PW, Higano CS, Shore ND, et al. Sipuleucel-T immunotherapy for castration-resistant prostate cancer. N Engl J Med 2010;363(5):411–22.
5. Cheever MA, Higano CS. PROVENGE (Sipuleucel-T) in prostate cancer: the first FDA-approved therapeutic cancer vaccine. Clin Cancer Res 2011;17(11): 3520–6.

6. Schwartzentruber DJ, Lawson DH, Richards JM, et al. gp100 peptide vaccine and interleukin-2 in patients with advanced melanoma. N Engl J Med 2011; 364(22):2119–27.

7. Schwartz RS. Paul Ehrlich's magic bullets. N Engl J Med 2004;350(11):1079–80.

8. Harbst K, Lauss M, Cirenajwis H, et al. Molecular and genetic diversity in the metastatic process of melanoma. J Pathol 2014;233(1):39–50.

9. Tosti G, di Pietro A, Ferrucci PF, et al. HSPPC-96 vaccine in metastatic melanoma patients: from the state of the art to a possible future. Expert Rev Vaccines 2009;8(11):1513–26.

10. Testori A, Richards J, Whitman E, et al. Phase III comparison of vitespen, an autologous tumor-derived heat shock protein gp96 peptide complex vaccine, with physician's choice of treatment for stage IV melanoma: the C-100–21 Study Group. J Clin Oncol 2008;26(6):955–62.

11. Tosti G, Cocorocchio E, Pennacchioli E, et al. Heat-shock proteins-based immunotherapy for advanced melanoma in the era of target therapies and immunomodulating agents. Expert Opin Biol Ther 2014;14(7):955–67.

12. Berd D, Sato T, Maguire H, et al. Immunopharmacologic analysis of an autologous, hapten-modified human melanoma vaccine. J Clin Oncol 2004;22(3): 403–15.

13. Berd D. M-Vax: an autologous, hapten-modified vaccine for human cancer. Expert Opin Biol Ther 2002;2(3):335–42.

14. Berd D. M-Vax: an autologous, hapten-modified vaccine for human cancer. Expert Rev Vaccines 2004;3(5):521–7.

15. Dillman RO, Nayak SK, Barth NM, et al. Clinical experience with autologous tumor cell lines for patient-specific vaccine therapy in metastatic melanoma. Cancer Biother Radiopharm 1998;13(3):165–76.

16. Dillman R, Selvan S, Schiltz P, et al. Phase I/II trial of melanoma patient-specific vaccine of proliferating autologous tumor cells, dendritic cells, and GM-CSF: planned interim analysis. Cancer Biother Radiopharm 2004;19(5):658–65.

17. Hersey P, Coates A, McCarthy W, et al. Adjuvant immunotherapy of patients with high-risk melanoma using vaccinia viral lysates of melanoma: results of a randomized trial. J Clin Oncol 2002;20:4148–90.

18. Suriano R, Rajoria S, George AL, et al. Follow-up analysis of a randomized phase III immunotherapeutic clinical trial on melanoma. Mol Clin Oncol 2013; 1(3):466–72.

19. Sondak V, Liu P, Tuthill R, et al. Adjuvant immunotherapy or resected, intermediate-thickness, node-negative melanoma with an allogeneic tumor vaccine: overall results of a randomized trial of the Southwest Oncology Group. J Clin Oncol 2002;20:2058–66.

20. Sosman J, Unger J, Liu P, et al. Adjuvant immunotherapy of resected, intermediate-thickness, node-negative melanoma with an allogeneic tumor vaccine: impact of HLA class I antigen expression on outcome. J Clin Oncol 2002; 20(8):2067–75.

21. Morton D, Hsueh E, Essner R, et al. Prolonged survival in patients receiving active immunotherapy with Canvaxin therapeutic vaccine after complete resection of melanoma metastatic to regional lymph nodes. Ann Surg 2002;236(4): 438–48.

22. Morton DL, Mozzillo N, Thompson JF, et al. An international, randomized, phase III trial of bacillus Calmette-Guerin (BCG) plus allogeneic melanoma vaccine (MCV) or placebo after compete resection of melanoma metastatic to regional or distant sites. J Clin Oncol 2007;25(18S) [abstract: 8508].

23. Morton D, Mozzillo N, Thompson J, et al. An international, randomized, double-blind, phase 3 study of the specific active immunotherapy agent, Onamelatucel-L (Canvaxin), compared to placebo as post-surgical adjuvant in AJCC stage IV melanoma. Ann Surg Oncol 2006;13(Suppl 2):5s.

24. Morton D, Ravindranath M, Irie R. Tumor gangliosides as targets for active specific immunotherapies of melanoma in man. In: Svennerholm L, Asbury A, Reisfeld R, et al, editors. Progress in brain research, vol. 104. Amsterdam: Elsevier; 1994. p. 251–75.

25. Kirkwood J, Ibrahim J, Sosman J, et al. High-dose interferon alpha 2b significantly prolongs relapse-free and overall survival compared with the GM2-KLH/QS-21 vaccine patients with resected stage IIB-III melanoma: results of intergroup trial E1694/S9512/C509801. J Clin Oncol 2001;19:2370.

26. Eggermont AM, Suciu S, Rutkowski P, et al. Adjuvant ganglioside GM2-KLH/QS-21 vaccination versus observation after resection of primary tumor >1.5 mm in patients with stage II melanoma: results of the EORTC 18961 randomized phase III trial. J Clin Oncol 2013;31(30):3831–7.

27. van der Bruggen P, Traversari C, Chomez P, et al. A gene encoding an antigen recognized by cytolytic T lymphocytes on a human melanoma. Science 1991; 254(5038):1643–7.

28. Rosenberg S, Yang J, Schwartzentruber D, et al. Immunologic and therapeutic evaluation of a synthetic peptide vaccine for the treatment of patients with metastatic melanoma. Nat Med 1998;4(3):321–7.

29. Hodi FS, O'Day SJ, McDermott DF, et al. Improved survival with ipilimumab in patients with metastatic melanoma. N Engl J Med 2010;363(8):711–23.

30. Lawson DH, Lee SJ, Tarhini AA, et al. E4697: phase III cooperative group study of yeast-derived granulocyte macrophage colony-stimulating factor (GM-CSF) versus placebo as adjuvant treatment of patients with completely resected stage III-IV melanoma. J Clin Oncol 2010;28(Suppl 15) [abstract: 8504].

31. Slingluff CL Jr, Petroni GR, Chianese-Bullock KA, et al. Randomized multicenter trial of the effects of melanoma-associated helper peptides and cyclophosphamide on the immunogenicity of a multipeptide melanoma vaccine. J Clin Oncol 2011;29(21):2924–32.

32. Rosenberg S, Yang J, Schwartzentruber D, et al. Impact of cytokine administration on the generation of antitumor reactivity in patients with metastatic melanoma receiving a peptide vaccine. J Immunol 1999;163:1690–5.

33. Slingluff CL Jr. The present and future of peptide vaccines for cancer: single or multiple, long or short, alone or in combination? Cancer J 2011;17(5):343–50.

34. Faries MB, Czerniecki BJ. Dendritic cells in melanoma immunotherapy. Curr Treat Options Oncol 2005;6(3):175–84.

35. Nestle F, Alijagic S, Gilliet M, et al. Vaccination of melanoma patients with peptide or tumor lysate-pulsed dendritic cells. Nat Med 1998;4(3):269–70.

36. Schadendorf D, Nestle F, Broecker E, et al. Dacarbacine (DTIC) versus vaccination with autologous peptide-pulsed dendritic cells as first-line treatment of patients with metastatic melanoma: results of a prospective-randomized phase III study. In: Grunberg SM, editor. American Society of Clinical Oncology, vol. 23. New Orleans (LA): American Society of Clinical Oncology; 2004. p. 709.

37. Zhou F, Ciric B, Zhang GX, et al. Immune tolerance induced by intravenous transfer of immature dendritic cells via up-regulating numbers of suppressive IL-10(+) IFN-gamma(+)-producing CD4(+) T cells. Immunol Res 2013; 56(1):1–8.

38. Palucka AK, Ueno H, Connolly J, et al. Dendritic cells loaded with killed alloge-neic melanoma cells can induce objective clinical responses and MART-1 spe-cific CD8+ T-cell immunity. J Immunother 2006;29(5):545–57.

39. Morton D, Eilber F, Holmes E, et al. BCG immunotherapy of malignant mela-noma: summary of a seven-year experience. Ann Surg 1974;180(4):635–43.

40. Sopkova B, Kolar V. Intralesional BCG application in malignant melanoma. Neoplasma 1976;23(4):421–6.

41. Mastrangelo M, Bellet R, Berkelhammer J, et al. Regression of pulmonary met-astatic disease associated with intralesional BCG therapy of intracutaneous melanoma metastases. Cancer 1975;36(4):1305–8.

42. McKhann CF, Hendrickson CG, Spitler LE, et al. Immunotherapy of melanoma with BCG: two fatalities following intralesional injection. Cancer 1975;35(2):514–20.

43. Sparks F, Silverstein M, Hunt J, et al. Complications of BCG immunotherapy in patients with cancer. N Engl J Med 1973;289:827–30.

44. Coit DG, Andtbacka R, Anker CJ, et al. Melanoma, version 2.2013: featured up-dates to the NCCN guidelines. J Natl Compr Canc Netw 2013;11(4):395–407.

45. Kidner TB, Morton DL, Lee DJ, et al. Combined intralesional bacille Calmette-Guerin (BCG) and topical imiquimod for in-transit melanoma. J Immunother 2012;35(9):716–20.

46. Hiniker SM, Chen DS, Knox SJ. Abscopal effect in a patient with melanoma. N Engl J Med 2012;366(21):2035 [author reply: 2035–6].

47. Kaufman HL, Bines SD. OPTIM trial: a phase III trial of an oncolytic herpes virus encoding GM-CSF for unresectable stage III or IV melanoma. Future Oncol 2010;6(6):941–9.

48. Senzer NN, Kaufman HL, Amatruda T, et al. Phase II clinical trial of a granulocyte-macrophage colony-stimulating factor-encoding, second-genera-tion oncolytic herpesvirus in patients with unresectable metastatic melanoma. J Clin Oncol 2009;27(34):5763–71.

49. Kaufman HL, Kim DW, DeRaffele G, et al. Local and distant immunity induced by intralesional vaccination with an oncolytic herpes virus encoding GM-CSF in pa-tients with stage IIIc and IV melanoma. Ann Surg Oncol 2009;17(3):718–30.

50. Andtbacka R, Collichio FA, Amatruda T, et al. OPTiM: a randomized phase III trial of talimogene laherparepvec (T-VEC) versus subcutaneous (SC) granulocyte-macrophage colony-stimulating factor (GM-CSF) for the treatment (tx) of unresected stage IIIB/C and IV melanoma. J Clin Oncol 2013;31(Suppl) [abstract: 9008].

51. Faries MB, Hsueh EC, Ye X, et al. Effect of granulocyte/macrophage colony-stimulating factor on vaccination with an allogeneic whole-cell melanoma vac-cine. Clin Cancer Res 2009;15(22):7029–35.

The Role of Radiation Therapy in Melanoma

Jacqueline Oxenberg, DO[a], John M. Kane III, MD[b],*

KEYWORDS

- Melanoma • Radiation therapy • Locoregional recurrence • Nodal metastases
- Lymphedema

KEY POINTS

- Adjuvant radiation therapy can reduce local recurrence for certain high-risk primary melanomas, including lentigo maligna, desmoplastic/neurotropic features, and mucosal melanomas (head and neck and anorectal).
- There are retrospective and limited prospective data to support adjuvant radiation following lymphadenectomy for nodal metastatic disease at high risk for regional recurrence.
- Radiation therapy is associated with increased potential toxicity, such as lower extremity lymphedema, and may negatively interact with concurrent adjuvant interferon therapy.

INTRODUCTION

Radiation therapy (RT) is a locoregional treatment that can be very effective at reducing the risk of recurrence for many cancers. Given that radiation is not tumor specific, there can also be significant toxicity to adjacent anatomic structures. Historically, melanoma was thought to be radiation "resistant." This assumption led to either its exclusion as an adjuvant therapy or very hypofractionated dosing regimens. More recent data would suggest that melanoma is radiation sensitive, including to standard fractionation treatment plans. This review examines high-risk situations for locoregional recurrence following melanoma surgical therapy, the available literature supporting the role of both adjuvant and definitive RT, and treatment-related complications. The use of RT for situations whereby melanoma is not typically treated surgically (uveal melanoma, brain metastases, palliation, and so forth) are not addressed.

[a] Department of Surgical Oncology, Roswell Park Cancer Institute, Elm and Carlton Streets, Buffalo, NY 14263, USA; [b] Melanoma-Sarcoma Service, Department of Surgical Oncology, Roswell Park Cancer Institute, Elm and Carlton Streets, Buffalo, NY 14263, USA
* Corresponding author.
E-mail address: john.kane@roswellpark.org

Surg Clin N Am 94 (2014) 1031–1047
http://dx.doi.org/10.1016/j.suc.2014.07.006
0039-6109/14/$ – see front matter © 2014 Elsevier Inc. All rights reserved.

surgical.theclinics.com

RADIATION FOR LOCAL CONTROL
Lentigo Maligna

Although it is only melanoma in situ, complete surgical excision of a lentigo maligna (LM) can be difficult secondary to the large size, poorly visualized margins, and cosmetically important locations such as the face. In addition, 16% to 50% of cases can have an associated invasive melanoma component (lentigo maligna melanoma [LMM]).[1–3] Local recurrence rates following conventional surgical resection can be as high as 20%.[4] However, even negative margin staged excisions or Mohs micrographic surgery with a low risk for local recurrence often produces a very morbid cutaneous defect.

In light of these issues, RT has been used as definitive therapy for LM. A small series by Harwood[5] reported on conventional fractionated RT for 17 patients with LM and 23 with LMM. The clinical response following RT took up to 24 months. Although the follow-up was variable, only 2 of the LM patients recurred, both of whom were salvaged by either surgery or additional radiation. Local control was obtained in 91% of the LMM patients. The 2 recurrences were both salvaged by surgical excision.

Grenz rays, or "soft" x-rays, are produced at low kilovoltages, being completely absorbed within the first 2 mm of the skin. Schmid-Wendtner and colleagues[6] examined 42 patients with LM and 22 with LMM treated with fractionated radiation (100 Gy). In contrast to the Harwood study, the nodular melanoma portion of the LMM lesion was excised before radiation. At a median follow-up of 15 months, local control was 100% in the LM group and 91% in the LMM patients (all recurrences were salvaged with surgery). Another study of Grenz rays/soft x-rays for definitive therapy involved patients with LM alone (n = 93), LMM (n = 54), or both components (n = 3).[7] The patients were older (mean age 70 years) and 90% of tumors were on the face. For patients with 2 years or more of follow-up, the local recurrence rate was only 5%. Eighty percent of recurrences were at the edge of the radiation field; all were salvaged with surgery or additional radiation. Only 2 patients developed nodal disease, both of whom died of distant metastases. The largest series of Grenz rays/soft x-rays for LM is 593 patients: definitive therapy in 350, partial excision/radiation in 71, and adjuvant therapy after surgery in 172.[8] The total radiation dose was 100 to 160 Gy (given as twice-weekly fractions over 3 weeks). Only 3.6% of patients with residual LM did not have a complete response, and the overall recurrence rate was only 9.8%. In most of the aforementioned studies, it was considered that the cosmetic outcome was very good, with only occasional radiation-field skin hypopigmentation or hyperpigmentation.

High-Risk Cutaneous Melanoma

Several primary tumor features, such as thickness, ulceration, anatomic location, and satellitosis, predict an increased risk for local recurrence. Reported local recurrence rates for melanomas greater than 4 mm are 12% to 13.2%.[9,10] Even melanomas 3 to 4 mm thick may recur up to 11.7%.[11] In 2 randomized, prospective trials of wide excision margins, ulceration was associated with a rate of local recurrence of 6.6% to 16.2%.[11,12] Local recurrence rates based on high-risk primary tumor site include 9.4% for head and neck, 11.1% for hands, and 11.6% for feet.[10,12] Many of these high-risk features are additive; the recurrence rate for ulcerated melanomas of the distal extremity or head and neck was the highest, at 16.2%.[12] Typically associated with thicker tumors, primary melanomas with histopathologic microsatellites have been shown to recur locally up to 14%.[13]

In 1983, Johanson and colleagues[14] reported on a very hypofractionated RT regimen (800 rad fractions × 3) for high-risk melanoma. There were 3 cohorts: 22

patients with microscopic residual tumor after surgery (3 primary tumor and 19 nodal), 9 patients with gross residual tumor after surgery (3 primary tumor and 6 nodal), and 23 patients with recurrent gross disease no longer amenable to surgical resection (including 15 with skin/subcutaneous tumor). Median follow-up was not specified, and 59% patients also received dacarbazine before the first and third doses of radiation. Only 1 of the 3 patients with primary tumor and positive margins recurred (14 months after radiation). At last follow-up, all 3 patients were alive and disease-free. Fifty-five percent of the patients with gross residual tumor had a complete response after radiation and there were no in-field recurrences. Finally, 39% of patients with unresectable gross disease also had a complete response, which was durable in 78%. There were also 5 postradiation partial responses and 3 patients with stable disease.

In a series by Stevens and colleagues[15] of postoperative RT for locally advanced melanoma, 32 patients received adjuvant radiation to the primary tumor site; 11 for a high-risk primary tumor and 21 after a previous recurrence. High-risk features included close or positive resection margins, satellitosis, or neurotropic/perineural features. Eighty-eight percent of tumors were on the head and neck. Hypofractionated regimens were used to a total dose of 30 to 36 Gy. Although not specifically calculated for each patient subset, the in-field recurrence rate for the entire study was only 11.5%. The 5-year overall survival for the high-risk primary tumors was 49%.

Desmoplastic and Neurotropic Melanoma

Representing only 1% to 4% of all melanoma cases, desmoplastic melanoma (DM) is most common in the head and neck region (37%–68%) and has an increased propensity for local recurrence.[16–20] Approximately 30% to 40% will also be neurotropic, with perineural invasion and extension along adjacent nerves.[21] Although one study showed no difference in local control between DM and case-matched controls, others have shown high local recurrence rates of 14% to 48% (including 27%–45% for the neurotropic variant).[16–19,22–24] Several studies have also shown that margin status and head and neck location are associated with an increased risk for local recurrence.[19,21,22,24,25]

Most of the published studies on adjuvant RT for DM are anecdotal in nature, but there are a few larger series. Vongtama and colleagues[20] identified 44 DM patients from their tumor registry, 21 with recurrent disease. Twenty-nine patients were treated with surgery alone, 1 received preoperative RT, and 14 underwent postoperative RT. Though not clearly stated, it appears that all of the patients who received radiation had recurrent tumor. Following initial surgery, the local recurrence rate was 48% with a median of 2 recurrences. The rate of subsequent local recurrence in 7 patients with a prior history of recurrence who did not receive RT was 57%. By contrast, there were no local recurrences in the patient group who received RT for a previous recurrence. There was no grade 3/4 toxicity (including the eye, ear, or bone). Foote and colleagues[26] noted a 91% 3-year local relapse-free survival in 24 DM patients who underwent surgery followed by adjuvant RT, including 71% with margins of less than 1 cm. The investigators stated that these findings were leading to the development of a randomized prospective trial. Finally, in a study by Chen and colleagues,[21] there was no significant difference in the local recurrence rate for 27 neurotropic DM patients who received 28 to 64 Gy of adjuvant RT in a comparison with 101 surgery-alone patients (7.4% vs 5.9%). However, the RT patients had significantly thicker tumors, a deeper Clark level, and narrower excision margins (60% ≤1 mm), placing them at a greater risk for local recurrence.

Head and Neck Mucosal Melanoma

Head and neck mucosal melanoma (nasal cavity and paranasal sinuses) is rare, accounting for only 1% of all melanoma. Negative margin wide excision is the potentially curative treatment, but is technically challenging because of the complex anatomic location and close proximity to critical structures. Local recurrences are common, ranging from 26% to 85%, and the mean time to local recurrence is 5 to 20 months.[27–30] Even with this locally aggressive biology, 5-year overall survival is still reasonable at 20% to 46%.[28–33] Consequently, RT has been studied as both postsurgical adjuvant therapy and definitive treatment.

There is significant variation in the postoperative adjuvant RT regimens used for head and neck mucosal melanoma from hypofractionation (6–8 Gy fractions × 3–5), total doses of 30 to 70 Gy, intensity-modulated RT (IMRT), and occasionally even combined photon/proton therapy.[29,30,34,35] Reported local control rates for postoperative RT following surgical resection have ranged from 29% to 83%.[29,34–37] Within the group of patients receiving adjuvant RT, Moreno and colleagues[30] found that cumulative doses of 54 Gy or greater resulted in better local control ($P = .02$).

Several retrospective studies have directly compared surgery alone with the addition of adjuvant RT. Owens and colleagues[36] reported a nonsignificant trend toward a lower rate of locoregional recurrence with adjuvant RT versus surgery alone (17% vs 45%; $P = .13$). Despite more locally advanced tumors in the 39 patients receiving postoperative RT, Temam and colleagues[37] found that local control was 62% as opposed to only 26% for the 30 patients in the surgery-alone group ($P = .02$). On Cox multivariate analysis, postoperative RT was a significant predictor of better local control (relative risk 0.4; $P = .05$). The largest retrospective review of adjuvant RT for head and neck mucosal melanoma is the GETTEC study of 160 patients from multiple institutions over 28 years.[33] Eighty-two patients who underwent surgery alone were compared with 78 patients who received postoperative RT. Although there was no difference in 5-year overall survival between the 2 groups (46% vs 27.5%, respectively; $P = .31$), the 5-year cumulative locoregional recurrence rate was significantly lower in the radiation group (29.9% vs 55.6%; $P<.01$). Most other series have also shown no difference in overall survival based on whether RT was administered.[30,33,36,37]

A few studies have specifically examined definitive RT, especially for the elderly or patients at high risk for harboring distant metastatic disease. In one series of 28 patients undergoing definitive RT, the initial complete response rate was 79% with a local control rate of 61% at the time of last follow-up/death.[38] Another study of 8 patients receiving 66 Gy of definitive IMRT had a 3-year local progression-free survival of 57.1% and a 3-year overall survival of 75%.[39] Wada and colleagues[40] reviewed 21 patients undergoing definitive RT and 10 patients who received adjuvant RT for gross residual tumor following surgical resection. There was an initial complete response rate of 29% and a partial response rate of 58%. The overall local recurrence rate was 41.9%. The investigators found that a dose per fraction of 3 Gy or more was associated with better local control ($P = .048$).

Despite the presence of adjacent aerodigestive and neurologic structures, RT for head and neck mucosal melanoma has been fairly well tolerated. Reported acute grade 2 to 3 toxicities include 15% to 39% skin, 19% to 61% mucosal, 6% to 11% salivary, and 12% ocular with late toxicities of 7% dermatitis, 6% mucositis, and 4% xerostomia.[30,35] Christopherson and colleagues[34] noted a 14% severe complication rate, including bilateral blindness and severe mucositis (all were associated with once-daily fractions). There are no reports of severe neurotoxicity (brain necrosis or myelopathy). Fatal complications, such as severe mucosal ulceration and uncontrolled hemorrhage, were rare at only 6.5%.[40]

Anorectal Melanoma

Anorectal melanoma (ARM) is exceedingly rare, but with a very high associated mortality secondary to early dissemination of distant metastatic disease. Although fairly morbid, ARM was historically treated with abdominoperineal resection (APR). However, most recent studies have shown no survival advantage for APR over local excision (LE).[41] In one study, although the rates of nodal relapse were similar for limited versus radical surgery (16.7 vs 15.4%; $P = .98$), local relapse risk was significantly higher (45.8% vs 0%; $P = .007$).[42] Consequently, RT has been used in an attempt to reduce the risk for local recurrence. In one small series from M.D. Anderson Cancer Center, 23 patients with ARM were treated with sphincter-sparing LE and inguinal lymph node dissection in 9 patients with nodal metastatic disease, followed by 30 Gy of hypofractionated RT.[43] Radiation was well tolerated, with self-limited radiation dermatitis in most patients, and only 17% developed late grade 2 proctitis. At a median follow-up of 32 months, the actuarial 5-year local control rate was 74% with a nodal control rate of 84%. No patients failed locoregionally as the only site of failure; therefore, salvage APR was not required. The conclusion was that sphincter-preserving LE with adjuvant RT is a low-morbidity alternative to APR with a comparable long-term outcome.

RADIATION FOR NODAL BASIN CONTROL
Risk Factors for Nodal Basin Recurrence

Regional lymphadenectomy is the potentially curative treatment for nodal metastatic melanoma. Owing to the proximity of major neurovascular structures to most anatomic lymph node basins, regional recurrence following lymphadenectomy can lead to significant morbidity (vascular occlusion, neuropathic pain, paralysis, skin ulceration, and bleeding). In the sentinel lymph node biopsy (SLNB) era, patients undergoing completion lymph node dissection (LND) typically have low nodal tumor burdens. Therefore, surgery alone is likely to be highly effective at obtaining regional control. By contrast, one would expect that bulky clinical nodal metastatic disease would be at higher risk for regional recurrence.

Several studies have attempted to define high-risk features for regional recurrence after melanoma lymphadenectomy. A small but early series by Monsour and colleagues[44] examined 48 patients who underwent LND for clinical nodal metastatic disease. The dissected nodal basin was 52% inguinal, 31% axillary, and 17% cervical. At a median follow-up of 24 months, nodal basin recurrence was 52%. On multivariate analysis, age older than 50 years was the only factor associated with an increased risk for recurrence (31% vs 66%; $P = .02$). Other features such as lymph node size, number of positive lymph nodes, extracapsular extension (ECE), and location of nodal basin were not significant. The presence of ECE did correlate with a more rapid recurrence (a median of 5 months vs 16 months for no ECE).

The largest study in the literature investigating patterns of relapse for nodal metastatic melanoma includes 1001 consecutive patients from M.D. Anderson Cancer Center.[45] Ninety-three percent of patients underwent LND for clinical disease, 64% had more than 1 positive lymph node, and only 1% of patients receive adjuvant nodal basin RT. The breakdown of involved nodal basin was 44% axillary, 29% cervical, 17% inguinal, and 10% ilioinguinal. All patients had a minimum follow-up of 10 years. The rate of recurrence after LND by nodal basin was 15% for cervical, 15% for axillary, and 17% for inguinal or ilioinguinal. The number of positive lymph nodes and ECE were the only factors independently associated with an increased risk for nodal basin recurrence. The recurrence rate was only 9% for 1 positive lymph node, but increased to 15% for 2 to 4, 17% for 5 to 10, and 33% for more than 10 ($P = .00001$). The risk for recurrence almost doubled for ECE; 28% versus 15% for no ECE ($P<.001$).

To determine a subset of patients that would potentially benefit from RT, Lee and colleagues[46] retrospectively assessed nodal basin recurrence following LND. Three hundred thirty-eight patients underwent a complete LND for metastatic melanoma; 75% were therapeutic and 25% were elective. The anatomic nodal basin was 47% axilla, 36% groin, and 17% cervical. The largest lymph node was at least 3 cm in 35% and 26% had 4 or more positive nodes. None of the patients underwent adjuvant RT, but 44% received adjuvant systemic therapy. At a median follow-up of 54 months, the estimated 10-year nodal basin failure rate was 30%. Several factors were predictive of nodal basin recurrence. Recurrence rates by lymph node size were 24% for less than 3 cm, 42% for 3 to 6 cm, and 80% for greater than 6 cm ($P<.001$). Increasing numbers of positive nodes also had a higher risk for recurrence; 25% for 1 to 3, 46% for 4 to 10, and 63% for more than 10 ($P = .0001$). On multivariate analysis, the anatomic nodal basin and ECE were significantly associated with nodal basin failure. The recurrence rate for cervical location was 43%, versus only 28% for axilla and 23% for groin ($P = .008$). The presence of ECE had an almost 3-fold higher risk for recurrence; 63% versus 23% ($P<.0001$). The investigators concluded that adjuvant nodal basin RT should be considered for cervical location, clinically involved/large nodes, ECE, and 4 or more nodes; they also suggested that clinical trials examining the role of adjuvant RT were warranted.

Based on the work of Lee and colleagues[46] and others, high-risk criteria for postlymphadenectomy nodal basin recurrence have been developed to stratify patients as potential candidates for adjuvant RT.[47] These guidelines take into account the interrelated risk factors of anatomic nodal basin, number of positive lymph nodes, size of the involved node, and ECE. A summary of standard high-risk criteria for postlymphadenectomy nodal basin recurrence is given in **Table 1**.

Adjuvant Radiation to Reduce Nodal Basin Recurrence

There have been a few single-treatment-arm retrospective institutional series, several retrospective comparative studies, one prospective phase II study, and only 2 randomized phase III trials examining adjuvant RT following melanoma LND. The results of these studies are summarized in **Table 2**. Although the single-arm studies all have

Table 1
High-risk criteria for nodal basin recurrence following lymphadenectomy for nodal metastatic melanoma

Basin	High-Risk Criteria
Cervical	>2 cm size *OR* >2 positive nodes *OR* ECE
Axilla	>3 cm size *OR* >4 positive nodes *OR* ECE
Epitrochlear	>3 cm size *OR* >4 positive nodes *OR* ECE
Inguinal	>3 cm size *AND* ECE >3 cm size *AND* >4 positive nodes >4 positive nodes *AND* ECE

Abbreviation: ECE, extracapsular extension.
From Agrawal S, Kane JM 3rd, Guadagnolo BA, et al. The benefits of adjuvant radiation therapy after therapeutic lymphadenectomy for clinically advanced, high-risk, lymph node metastatic melanoma. Cancer 2009;115(24):5836–44; with permission.

Table 2
Selected published studies of regional control for adjuvant radiation therapy following lymph node dissection for nodal metastatic melanoma

Authors,[Ref.] Year	Type	Nodal Basin	Number of Patients RT	No RT	RT Dose (Gy)	Median F/U (mo)	Regional Control Rate RT (%)	No RT (%)	P Value	
Adjuvant Radiation										
Ballo et al,[58] 2003	Retro	C	160		30	78	94			[10 y]
Ballo et al,[64] 2002	Retro	A	89		30	63	87			[5 y]
Ballo et al,[59] 2004	Retro	I	40		30	22.5	74			[3 y]
Burmeister et al,[51] 2006	Pro	C, A, I	234		48	58.4	91			[5 y]
Adjuvant Radiation vs LND Alone										
Moncrieff et al,[48] 2008	Retro	C	129	587	33	34.7	89.9	93.9	.20	[6 y]
Strojan et al,[49] 2010	Retro	C	43	40	60	25	78	56	.015	[2 y]
Pinkham et al,[50] 2013	Retro	A	121	156	48	23	86	87		[2 y]
Gojkovic-Horvat et al,[65] 2012	Retro	I	37	64	50.6		86	91	.395	[2 y]
Bibault et al,[60] 2011	Retro	C, A, I	60	26	50	73	C 85 A 90 I 80	50 70 72	.4	
Agrawal et al,[52] 2009	Retro	C, A, I	509	106	30	60	89.8	59.4	<.0001	[5 y]
Creagan et al,[53] 1978	Pro		27	29	50		88.9	96.6		
Burmeister et al,[54] 2012	Pro	C, A, I	109	108	48	40	81	69	.041	[3 y]

Abbreviations: A, axillary; C, cervical; F/U, follow-up; I, inguinal; LND, lymph node dissection; mo, months; Pro, prospective; Retro, retrospective; RT, radiation therapy; y, year.

impressive regional control rates following adjuvant RT, the potential benefit of RT in the comparative studies is less clear. To better understand these conflicting and controversial findings, the details of many of the published series need to be closely scrutinized. The larger prospective studies also deserve discussion in depth.

All of the single-arm studies included only melanoma patients that were truly considered to be at high risk for regional recurrence after LND (multiple positive lymph nodes, enlarged nodes, ECE, or recurrent disease). Consequently, regional control exceeding 90% would be considered superior to expected historical recurrence rates. By contrast, many of the retrospective comparative studies compared the high-risk patients receiving adjuvant RT with a more general low-risk population undergoing lymphadenectomy alone. Therefore, there is significant retrospective treatment selection bias whereby only the patients at very high risk for regional recurrence were administered RT. In the study by Moncrieff and colleagues,[48] macroscopic nodal disease (P<.0001) and the need for radical neck dissection and/or parotidectomy (P<.0001) were significantly more likely to receive RT. However, there was no difference in regional recurrence when an attempt was made to stratify by N status (N 1–3). Patients receiving adjuvant cervical RT in the study by Strojan and colleagues[49] were significantly more likely to have ECE (P = .026), a higher N stage (P = .003), and a higher risk-factor score (P<.0001). Despite this major imbalance in risk factors in favor of surgery alone, the adjuvant RT patients still had a significantly higher regional recurrence-free survival. On multivariate analysis, risk-factor score and adjuvant RT (hazard ratio [HR] 6.3, 95% confidence interval [CI] 2.0–20.6; P = .002) were both associated with improved regional control. Although there was no formal statistical analysis of baseline patient characteristics in the study by Pinkham and colleagues,[50] there were obvious differences between patients who received adjuvant axillary RT versus surgery alone in terms of 4 or more positive nodes (39% vs 15%), 4 cm or larger size (52% vs 16%), and ECE (81% vs 38%). There was also a complex scoring system for regional recurrence, such as in-field versus adjacent field and nodal versus dermal versus scar. On univariate analysis, adjuvant RT was associated with a much lower risk for in-field nodal recurrence (odds ratio [OR] 0.19; P = .01), but a significantly higher risk for adjacent field recurrence (OR 4.27; P = .02). This latter finding was likely secondary to more aggressive tumor biology in the patients who received RT.

In 2006, the Trans Tasmanian Radiation Oncology Group (TROG) published the results of their multicenter prospective phase II study of adjuvant postoperative RT following melanoma nodal surgery.[51] Two hundred thirty patients received 45 to 50 Gy of adjuvant RT to the cervical region (33%), axilla (44%), or ilioinguinal basin (20%). Patients were at high risk for regional recurrence; 51% had 3 or more positive nodes and 75% had ECE. The in-field relapse rate was only 6.8% with an adjacent relapse rate of 13.6%. The regional control curve for the entire cohort is shown in **Fig. 1**. No factors (known vs unknown primary, nodal basin site, number of positive nodes, ECE, or number of operations) were associated with regional control.

The largest retrospective comparative study of adjuvant RT for high-risk nodal metastatic melanoma is by Agrawal and colleagues.[52] Data were collected on 615 melanoma patients undergoing therapeutic lymphadenectomy from 2 tertiary cancer centers. All patients were at high risk for regional recurrence based on previously described risk factors (number of positive nodes, lymph node size, and ECE). Capitalizing on preexisting institutional treatment biases, 106 patients who underwent LND alone were compared with 509 who also received adjuvant RT. As shown in **Fig. 2**, there was a significant improvement in regional control with the addition of adjuvant RT. On multivariate analysis, primary tumor thickness up to 4 mm versus greater than 4 mm (P = .0004), number of positive lymph nodes up to 3 versus 4 or more

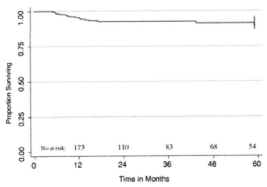

Fig. 1. Regional control following adjuvant radiation therapy for 230 patients enrolled in the Trans Tasmanian Radiation Oncology Group prospective phase II trial 96.06. (*From* Burmeister BH, Mark Smithers B, Burmeister E, et al. A prospective phase II study of adjuvant postoperative radiation therapy following nodal surgery in malignant melanoma-Trans Tasman Radiation Oncology Group (TROG) Study 96.06. Radiother Oncol 2006;81(2):136–42; with permission.)

(*P* = .0015), number of lymph nodes removed up to 14 versus 15 or more (*P* = .01), and adjuvant RT (*P*<.0001) were associated with improved regional control. ECE and lymph node size were not significant. Interestingly, the 5-year disease-specific survival was also significantly higher following adjuvant RT (51% vs 30%; *P*<.0001). This intriguing result was difficult to explain, even when accounting for the retrospective, nonrandomized nature of the study.

The first prospective, randomized study of adjuvant RT for nodal metastatic melanoma was published by Creagan and colleagues[53] in 1978. Unfortunately, this study was very small, there is no mention of the nodal basins involved, and, although the regional recurrences are described, no statistical analysis was performed. Therefore, the only prospective, randomized phase III trial specifically assessing the impact of adjuvant RT on regional recurrence for nodal metastatic melanoma is by the Australian and New Zealand Melanoma Trials Group/TROG.[54] Based on the previous TROG 96.06 prospective phase II trial, patients with high-risk nodal metastatic melanoma were randomized 1:1 to LND alone or 48 Gy of adjuvant RT within 12 weeks of lymphadenectomy. High risk was defined as at least 1 of the following features; 1 or more positive parotid nodes, 2 or more positive cervical or axillary nodes, 3 or more positive inguinal nodes, cervical node larger than 3 cm, axillary or inguinal node larger than 4 cm, or ECE. There were 108 eligible patients in the surgery-alone group versus 109 patients in the adjuvant RT group. Both cohorts were evenly matched in terms of baseline characteristics. The axilla was the most common nodal basin at 41%, 39% to 41% had a lymph node larger than 4 cm, approximately half of the patients had ECE, and no more than 5% received adjuvant interferon. At a median follow-up of 40 months, the 3-year cumulative rate of lymph node field recurrence was significantly higher in the surgery-alone group at 31%, compared with 19% for the adjuvant RT group (HR 0.56, 95% CI 0.32–0.98; *P* = .041). The lymph node field relapse curves are shown in **Fig. 3**. In contrast to the findings of Agrawal and colleagues,[52] there was no difference in survival between the 2 cohorts.

Three novel approaches to RT for nodal metastatic disease deserve brief mention. In a study by Foote and colleagues,[55] 12 patients with bulky lymph node metastases received 48 Gy (in 20 fractions) of preoperative RT. The clinical partial response rate was 58%. Completion LND was performed in 10 patients with a minor wound

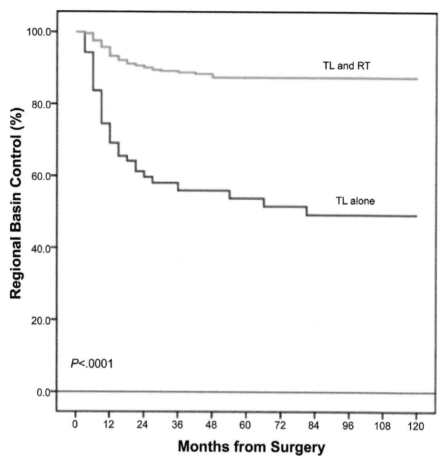

Fig. 2. Regional lymph node basin control following therapeutic lymphadenectomy alone compared with therapeutic lymphadenectomy with adjuvant radiation therapy for clinically advanced nodal metastatic melanoma. RT, radiation therapy; TL, therapeutic lymphadenectomy. (*From* Agrawal S, Kane JM 3rd, Guadagnolo BA, et al. The benefits of adjuvant radiation therapy after therapeutic lymphadenectomy for clinically advanced, high-risk, lymph node metastatic melanoma. Cancer 2009;115(24):5836–44; with permission.)

complication rate of only 40%. Although the follow-up was short, the 1-year in-field control rate was 92%. Ballo and colleagues[56] reported on 36 patients with clinical cervical nodal metastatic melanoma who underwent surgical excision of only the clinical disease followed by 30 Gy of hypofractionated radiation in lieu of a formal completion LND. The median number of lymph nodes removed was 1 (range 1–8), median number of positive nodes was 1 (range 1–3), and median lymph node size was 2 cm. At a median follow-up of 63 months, the 5-year actuarial regional control rate was 93%. The investigators concluded that regional RT may play a role in patients for whom observation of the remaining cervical lymph nodes is being considered based on medical comorbidities or an anticipated low residual nodal tumor burden. A similar study by Bonnen and colleagues[57] reported on the long-term results of an M.D. Anderson Cancer Center protocol of elective RT to both the primary tumor site and the ipsilateral regional lymph node basin for high-risk primary cutaneous head and neck melanomas. One hundred fifty-seven patients with stage I/II primary head and neck melanoma

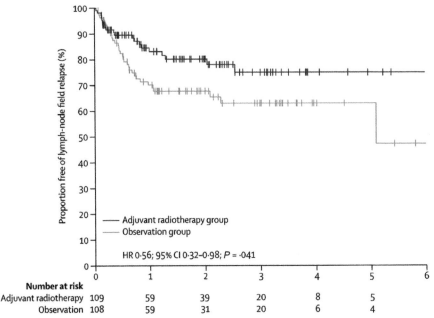

Fig. 3. Kaplan- Meier curve for lymph node field relapse for patients receiving adjuvant radiation therapy versus observation following lymphadenectomy for nodal metastatic melanoma in the Australian and New Zealand Melanoma Trials Group/TROG prospective randomized phase III trial. CI, confidence interval; HR, hazard ratio. (*From* Burmeister BH, Henderson MA, Ainslie J, et al. Adjuvant radiotherapy vs observation alone for patients at risk of lymph-node field relapse after therapeutic lymphadenectomy for melanoma: a randomised trial. Lancet Oncol 2012;13(6):589–9; with permission.)

either at least 1.5 mm thick or at least Clark level IV underwent only wide excision of the primary tumor site followed by 30 Gy hypofractionated RT. At a median follow-up of 68 months, the 10-year actuarial locoregional control rate was 86% with a disease-specific survival of 58% and an overall survival of 22%. Only 6% of patients developed symptomatic treatment-related complications. The investigators suggested that elective regional nodal basin RT could be an alternative to SLNB or performing a completion LND after a positive SLNB in certain patients.

Morbidity of Adjuvant Nodal Basin Radiation

Given that axillary or inguinal lymphadenectomy alone can produce extremity lymphedema, there has been concern that adjuvant nodal basin RT would increase this risk. In addition, many of the melanoma RT regimens are hypofractionated, resulting in a greater potential for late toxicity. This risk for late toxicity is partially counterbalanced by the fact that long-term survival in patients with bulky nodal metastatic disease is limited. Consequently, the available data have been mixed in terms of the toxicity of adjuvant nodal basin RT.

General morbidity

The most common early radiation toxicity in the randomized phase III trial was dermatitis, especially the axilla (17%).[54] The rate of other toxicities (seroma, wound infection, pain) was very low and there was no difference between the RT and observation groups. In most studies, general grade 2 late radiation toxicity ranges from 10% to

45%.[52,58–60] Uncommon nonlymphedema toxicities include mucositis, chronic skin fibrosis, subcutaneous or bone/joint changes, and nerve injury. Agrawal and colleagues[52] found that the 5-year cumulative overall morbidity was significantly higher for adjuvant RT than for surgery alone (20% vs 13%; P = .004). However, many studies have shown that there are also significant variations in the toxicity patterns based on the specific nodal basin being irradiated.

Cervical basin morbidity

Following cervical RT, the more common grade 2/3 toxicities from the TROG prospective phase II trial were skin changes (22%), subcutaneous changes (10%), mucositis (5%), and nerve/spinal cord injury (2%).[61] Reported rare complications include ipsilateral hearing loss, hypothyroidism, dysphagia, and xerostomia.[58,62] Strojan and colleagues[49] showed that late toxicity was significantly higher following adjuvant RT in comparison with surgery alone (27.8% vs 17.7%; P<.05). Toxicity did not correlate with the extent of surgery, the total RT dose, or the individual fraction dose. Conversely, other studies have shown no difference in toxicity following the addition of cervical RT.[60] One small series of 13 patients who received adjuvant bilateral cervical RT for nodal metastatic melanoma noted that the overall complication rate was 56% with a median survival of only 9 months.[62] The investigators concluded that the high toxicity of bilateral RT was not justified in light of the associated dismal prognosis.

Axillary basin morbidity

Late grade 2/3 skin changes (11%), subcutaneous changes (5%), and bone joint changes (2%) are fairly uncommon following adjuvant axillary RT.[61] However, Bibault and colleagues[60] found that RT significantly increased the risk for grade 2 toxicity in comparison with surgery alone (P = .047). Rare complications of adjuvant axillary RT include brachial plexopathy, rib fracture, and transient pneumonitis.[63] One study compared hypofractionated adjuvant axillary RT using a standard axillary field (95 patients) with an extended field that included the supraclavicular fossa (105 patients).[63] There was no difference in 5-year nodal basin control (89% vs 86%, respectively; P = .4), but complications were significantly higher for the extended field (39%) than the standard axillary field (27%) (P = .047).

Interestingly the reported rates for major lymphedema (grade 2/3) following adjuvant axillary RT are surprisingly low, at 7% to 21%.[51,52,60,61,63] Ballo and colleagues[64] noted a postaxillary RT 5-year actuarial lymphedema-free survival (any grade) of 57%. On univariate analysis, the number of lymph nodes removed, RT dose, and field size were not associated with the risk for lymphedema.

Ilioinguinal basin morbidity

The ilioinguinal basin has been the most problematic in terms of adjuvant RT toxicity. Major late skin and subcutaneous tissue changes are seen in 21% to 30% of patients (including 3% grade 4 toxicity).[61] Up to 5% of patients will have post-RT wound-healing issues requiring surgical intervention.[59] However, one study did not find a statistically significant difference in general grade 2 toxicity for ilioinguinal lymphadenectomy with or without adjuvant RT.[60]

Unfortunately, the risk for moderate to severe post-RT lower extremity lymphedema is fairly significant, at 18% to 44%.[52,59,61,65] Given that lymphedema is not uncommon after ilioinguinal LND alone, it is somewhat difficult to determine the contribution of the adjuvant RT to this problem. Ballo and colleagues[59] found that 50% of patients undergoing adjuvant ilioinguinal RT had grade 2 lymphedema before the start of radiation. Although there was increased lower extremity lymphedema following adjuvant RT in the study by Gojkovic-Horvat and colleagues[65] (40.7% for radiation vs 29.2% for surgery alone), this difference was not statistically significant ($P = .321$). Both of these studies also showed trends toward an increased risk for post-RT lymphedema when the patient's body mass index was greater than 25 kg/m^2.

Morbidity of adjuvant interferon and radiation

The same high-risk features that would make a melanoma patient a potential candidate for adjuvant nodal basin RT would also predict a high risk for harboring occult distant metastatic disease. Therefore, many of these patients would be considered candidates for adjuvant interferon therapy. As there are preclinical data to support that interferon can act as a radiosensitizer, there are several small case series suggesting that adjuvant interferon-α2b therapy, either concurrent with or temporally in close proximity to adjuvant RT, might potentiate radiation toxicity. Two studies have shown that radiation-related complications occurred in 50% of patients receiving interferon/adjuvant RT.[66,67] Many of the grade 3 complications involved skin or soft tissue (mucositis, moist desquamation, necrosis, severe fibrosis, or delayed wound healing). However, there were also some very rare and unexpected radiation toxicities in this population, namely severe pneumonitis, myelitis, and radiation brain necrosis.[66–68] Although these findings are anecdotal, given that there is no urgency to administer adjuvant interferon, it would be prudent to consider delaying the initiation of interferon therapy until at least 30 days after the completion of RT.

SUMMARY

Many of the indications for adjuvant RT mentioned herein also place a melanoma patient at very high risk for harboring distant metastatic disease. Consequently, some have argued that RT would be of limited value in a cohort with such a dismal long-term prognosis. Others have cited the lack of an overall survival benefit as an additional reason to not consider RT. However, the 5-year survival for most high-risk melanoma situations is still 18% to 75%.[1,15,16,27,30,33–37,42,43,51,58,64,69] This figure would be comparable with or superior to many other primary cancers for which RT is considered to improve locoregional control (esophagus, gastric, pancreas). In addition, the morbidity of recurrent melanoma in the head and neck region, a previously dissected nodal basin, or the anorectum is significant. Therefore, the decision to consider adjuvant RT for high-risk melanoma should be individualized based on the predicted risk for locoregional recurrence and its implications, counterbalanced by the potential associated treatment toxicity and anticipated life expectancy.

REFERENCES

1. Agarwal-Antal N, Bowen GM, Gerwels JW. Histologic evaluation of lentigo maligna with permanent sections: implications regarding current guidelines. J Am Acad Dermatol 2002;47(5):743–8.
2. Megahed M, Schon M, Selimovic D, et al. Reliability of diagnosis of melanoma in situ. Lancet 2002;359(9321):1921–2.
3. Wayte DM, Helwig EB. Melanotic freckle of Hutchinson. Cancer 1968;21(5): 893–911.
4. Osborne JE, Hutchinson PE. A follow-up study to investigate the efficacy of initial treatment of lentigo maligna with surgical excision. Br J Plast Surg 2002; 55(8):611–5.
5. Harwood AR. Conventional fractionated radiotherapy for 51 patients with lentigo maligna and lentigo maligna melanoma. Int J Radiat Oncol Biol Phys 1983;9(7): 1019–21.

6. Schmid-Wendtner MH, Brunner B, Konz B, et al. Fractionated radiotherapy of lentigo maligna and lentigo maligna melanoma in 64 patients. J Am Acad Dermatol 2000;43(3):477–82.

7. Farshad A, Burg G, Panizzon R, et al. A retrospective study of 150 patients with lentigo maligna and lentigo maligna melanoma and the efficacy of radiotherapy using Grenz or soft X-rays. Br J Dermatol 2002;146(6):1042–6.

8. Hedblad MA, Mallbris L. Grenz ray treatment of lentigo maligna and early lentigo maligna melanoma. J Am Acad Dermatol 2012;67(1):60–8.

9. Heaton KM, Sussman JJ, Gershenwald JE, et al. Surgical margins and prognostic factors in patients with thick (>4 mm) primary melanoma. Ann Surg Oncol 1998;5(4):322–8.

10. Urist MM, Balch CM, Soong S, et al. The influence of surgical margins and prognostic factors predicting the risk of local recurrence in 3445 patients with primary cutaneous melanoma. Cancer 1985;55(6):1398–402.

11. Karakousis CP, Balch CM, Urist MM, et al. Local recurrence in malignant melanoma: long-term results of the multiinstitutional randomized surgical trial. Ann Surg Oncol 1996;3(5):446–52.

12. Balch CM, Soong SJ, Smith T, et al. Long-term results of a prospective surgical trial comparing 2 cm vs. 4 cm excision margins for 740 patients with 1-4 mm melanomas. Ann Surg Oncol 2001;8(2):101–8.

13. Kelly JW, Sagebiel RW, Calderon W, et al. The frequency of local recurrence and microsatellites as a guide to reexcision margins for cutaneous malignant melanoma. Ann Surg 1984;200(6):759–63.

14. Johanson CR, Harwood AR, Cummings BJ, et al. 0-7-21 Radiotherapy in nodular melanoma. Cancer 1983;51(2):226–32.

15. Stevens G, Thompson JF, Firth I, et al. Locally advanced melanoma: results of postoperative hypofractionated radiation therapy. Cancer 2000;88(1):88–94.

16. Quinn MJ, Crotty KA, Thompson JF, et al. Desmoplastic and desmoplastic neurotropic melanoma: experience with 280 patients. Cancer 1998;83(6):1128–35.

17. Smithers BM, McLeod GR, Little JH. Desmoplastic melanoma: patterns of recurrence. World J Surg 1992;16(2):186–90.

18. Livestro DP, Muzikansky A, Kaine EM, et al. Biology of desmoplastic melanoma: a case-control comparison with other melanomas. J Clin Oncol 2005;23(27):6739–46.

19. Smithers BM, McLeod GR, Little JH. Desmoplastic, neural transforming and neurotropic melanoma: a review of 45 cases. Aust N Z J Surg 1990;60(12):967–72.

20. Vongtama R, Safa A, Gallardo D, et al. Efficacy of radiation therapy in the local control of desmoplastic malignant melanoma. Head Neck 2003;25(6):423–8.

21. Chen JY, Hruby G, Scolyer RA, et al. Desmoplastic neurotropic melanoma: a clinicopathologic analysis of 128 cases. Cancer 2008;113(10):2770–8.

22. Posther KE, Selim MA, Mosca PJ, et al. Histopathologic characteristics, recurrence patterns, and survival of 129 patients with desmoplastic melanoma. Ann Surg Oncol 2006;13(5):728–39.

23. Egbert B, Kempson R, Sagebiel R. Desmoplastic malignant melanoma. A clinicohistopathologic study of 25 cases. Cancer 1988;62(9):2033–41.

24. Jaroszewski DE, Pockaj BA, DiCaudo DJ, et al. The clinical behavior of desmoplastic melanoma. Am J Surg 2001;182(6):590–5.

25. Maurichi A, Miceli R, Camerini T, et al. Pure desmoplastic melanoma: a melanoma with distinctive clinical behavior. Ann Surg 2010;252(6):1052–7.

26. Foote MC, Burmeister B, Burmeister E, et al. Desmoplastic melanoma: the role of radiotherapy in improving local control. ANZ J Surg 2008;78(4):273–6.
27. Bridger AG, Smee D, Baldwin MA, et al. Experience with mucosal melanoma of the nose and paranasal sinuses. ANZ J Surg 2005;75(4):192–7.
28. Huang S-, Liao C-, Kan C, et al. Primary mucosal melanoma of the nasal cavity and paranasal sinuses: 12 Years of experience. J Otolaryngol 2007;36(2):124–9.
29. Kingdom TT, Kaplan MJ. Mucosal melanoma of the nasal cavity and paranasal sinuses. Head Neck 1995;17(3):184–9.
30. Moreno MA, Roberts DB, Kupferman ME, et al. Mucosal melanoma of the nose and paranasal sinuses, a contemporary experience from the M. D. Anderson Cancer Center. Cancer 2010;116(9):2215–23.
31. Chan RC, Chan JY, Wei WI. Mucosal melanoma of the head and neck: 32-year experience in a tertiary referral hospital. Laryngoscope 2012;122(12):2749–53.
32. Narasimhan K, Kucuk O, Lin HS, et al. Sinonasal mucosal melanoma: a 13-year experience at a single institution. Skull Base 2009;19(4):255–62.
33. Benlyazid A, Thariat J, Temam S, et al. Postoperative radiotherapy in head and neck mucosal melanoma: a GETTEC study. Arch Otolaryngol Head Neck Surg 2010;136(12):1219–25.
34. Christopherson K, Malyapa RS, Werning JW, et al. Radiation therapy for mucosal melanoma of the head and neck. Am J Clin Oncol 2013. [Epub ahead of print].
35. Wu AJ, Gomez J, Zhung JE, et al. Radiotherapy after surgical resection for head and neck mucosal melanoma. Am J Clin Oncol 2010;33(3):281–5.
36. Owens JM, Roberts DB, Myers JN. The role of postoperative adjuvant radiation therapy in the treatment of mucosal melanomas of the head and neck region. Arch Otolaryngol Head Neck Surg 2003;129(8):864–8.
37. Temam S, Mamelle G, Marandas P, et al. Postoperative radiotherapy for primary mucosal melanoma of the head and neck. Cancer 2005;103(2):313–9.
38. Gilligan D, Slevin NJ. Radical radiotherapy for 28 cases of mucosal melanoma in the nasal cavity and sinuses. Br J Radiol 1991;64(768):1147–50.
39. Combs SE, Konkel S, Thilmann C, et al. Local high-dose radiotherapy and sparing of normal tissue using intensity-modulated radiotherapy (IMRT) for mucosal melanoma of the nasal cavity and paranasal sinuses. Strahlenther Onkol 2007;183(2):63–8.
40. Wada H, Nemoto K, Ogawa Y, et al. A multi-institutional retrospective analysis of external radiotherapy for mucosal melanoma of the head and neck in Northern Japan. Int J Radiat Oncol Biol Phys 2004;59(2):495–500.
41. Yap LB, Neary P. A comparison of wide local excision with abdominoperineal resection in anorectal melanoma. Melanoma Res 2004;14(2):147–50.
42. Belli F, Gallino GF, Lo Vullo S, et al. Melanoma of the anorectal region: the experience of the National Cancer Institute of Milano. Eur J Surg Oncol 2009;35(7):757–62.
43. Ballo MT, Gershenwald JE, Zagars GK, et al. Sphincter-sparing local excision and adjuvant radiation for anal-rectal melanoma. J Clin Oncol 2002;20(23):4555–8.
44. Monsour PD, Sause WT, Avent JM, et al. Local control following therapeutic nodal dissection for melanoma. J Surg Oncol 1993;54(1):18–22.
45. Calabro A, Singletary SE, Balch CM. Patterns of relapse in 1001 consecutive patients with melanoma nodal metastases. Arch Surg 1989;124(9):1051–5.
46. Lee RJ, Gibbs JF, Proulx GM, et al. Nodal basin recurrence following lymph node dissection for melanoma: implications for adjuvant radiotherapy. Int J Radiat Oncol Biol Phys 2000;46(2):467–74.

47. Ballo MT, Ross MI, Cormier JN, et al. Combined-modality therapy for patients with regional nodal metastases from melanoma. Int J Radiat Oncol Biol Phys 2006;64(1):106–13.

48. Moncrieff MD, Martin R, O'Brien CJ, et al. Adjuvant postoperative radiotherapy to the cervical lymph nodes in cutaneous melanoma: is there any benefit for high-risk patients? Ann Surg Oncol 2008;15(11):3022–7.

49. Strojan P, Jancar B, Cemazar M, et al. Melanoma metastases to the neck nodes: role of adjuvant irradiation. Int J Radiat Oncol Biol Phys 2010;77(4):1039–45.

50. Pinkham MB, Foote MC, Burmeister E, et al. Stage III melanoma in the axilla: patterns of regional recurrence after surgery with and without adjuvant radiation therapy. Int J Radiat Oncol Biol Phys 2013;86(4):702–8.

51. Burmeister BH, Mark Smithers B, Burmeister E, et al. A prospective phase II study of adjuvant postoperative radiation therapy following nodal surgery in malignant melanoma-Trans Tasman Radiation Oncology Group (TROG) Study 96.06. Radiother Oncol 2006;81(2):136–42.

52. Agrawal S, Kane JM 3rd, Guadagnolo BA, et al. The benefits of adjuvant radiation therapy after therapeutic lymphadenectomy for clinically advanced, high-risk, lymph node-metastatic melanoma. Cancer 2009;115(24):5836–44.

53. Creagan ET, Cupps RE, Ivins JC, et al. Adjuvant radiation therapy for regional nodal metastases from malignant melanoma: a randomized, prospective study. Cancer 1978;42(5):2206–10.

54. Burmeister BH, Henderson MA, Ainslie J, et al. Adjuvant radiotherapy versus observation alone for patients at risk of lymph-node field relapse after therapeutic lymphadenectomy for melanoma: a randomised trial. Lancet Oncol 2012; 13(6):589–97.

55. Foote M, Burmeister B, Dwyer P, et al. An innovative approach for locally advanced stage III cutaneous melanoma: radiotherapy, followed by nodal dissection. Melanoma Res 2012;22(3):257–62.

56. Ballo MT, Garden AS, Myers JN, et al. Melanoma metastatic to cervical lymph nodes: can radiotherapy replace formal dissection after local excision of nodal disease? Head Neck 2005;27(8):718–21.

57. Bonnen MD, Ballo MT, Myers JN, et al. Elective radiotherapy provides regional control for patients with cutaneous melanoma of the head and neck. Cancer 2004;100(2):383–9.

58. Ballo MT, Bonnen MD, Garden AS, et al. Adjuvant irradiation for cervical lymph node metastases from melanoma. Cancer 2003;97(7):1789–96.

59. Ballo MT, Zagars GK, Gershenwald JE, et al. A critical assessment of adjuvant radiotherapy for inguinal lymph node metastases from melanoma. Ann Surg Oncol 2004;11(12):1079–84.

60. Bibault JE, Dewas S, Mirabel X, et al. Adjuvant radiation therapy in metastatic lymph nodes from melanoma. Radiat Oncol 2011;6:12.

61. Burmeister BH, Smithers BM, Davis S, et al. Radiation therapy following nodal surgery for melanoma: an analysis of late toxicity. ANZ J Surg 2002;72(5):344–8.

62. Guadagnolo BA, Myers JN, Zagars GK. Role of postoperative irradiation for patients with bilateral cervical nodal metastases from cutaneous melanoma: a critical assessment. Head Neck 2010;32(6):708–13.

63. Beadle BM, Guadagnolo BA, Ballo MT, et al. Radiation therapy field extent for adjuvant treatment of axillary metastases from malignant melanoma. Int J Radiat Oncol Biol Phys 2009;73(5):1376–82.

64. Ballo MT, Strom EA, Zagars GK, et al. Adjuvant irradiation for axillary metastases from malignant melanoma. Int J Radiat Oncol Biol Phys 2002;52(4):964–72.

65. Gojkovic-Horvat A, Jancar B, Blas M, et al. Adjuvant radiotherapy for palpable melanoma metastases to the groin: when to irradiate? Int J Radiat Oncol Biol Phys 2012;83(1):310–6.
66. Hazard LJ, Sause WT, Noyes RD. Combined adjuvant radiation and interferon-alpha 2B therapy in high-risk melanoma patients: the potential for increased radiation toxicity. Int J Radiat Oncol Biol Phys 2002;52(3):796–800.
67. Gyorki DE, Ainslie J, Joon ML, et al. Concurrent adjuvant radiotherapy and interferon-alpha2b for resected high risk stage III melanoma – a retrospective single centre study. Melanoma Res 2004;14(3):223–30.
68. Conill C, Jorcano S, Domingo-Domenech J, et al. Toxicity of combined treatment of adjuvant irradiation and interferon alpha2b in high-risk melanoma patients. Melanoma Res 2007;17(5):304–9.
69. Thariat J, Poissonnet G, Marcy PY, et al. Effect of surgical modality and hypo-fractionated split-course radiotherapy on local control and survival from sino-nasal mucosal melanoma. Clin Oncol (R Coll Radiol) 2011;23(9):579–86.

Indications and Options for Systemic Therapy in Melanoma

Vernon K. Sondak, MD[a,b,*], Geoffrey T. Gibney, MD[a,b]

KEYWORDS

- Melanoma • Immunotherapy • Targeted therapy • Adjuvant therapy

KEY POINTS

- Adjuvant therapy after resection of high-risk melanoma remains suboptimal.
- Regular and pegylated interferon alfa may reduce recurrence rates and impact survival, but the hope is that newer agents may provide better survival impact with less toxicity.
- Immunotherapy for metastatic melanoma has advanced substantially.
- The discovery of driver mutations, such as the *BRAF* V600E mutation, has led to the development of new molecularly targeted therapies.
- Combination therapy involving molecularly targeted agents shows great promise and is being actively tested in clinical trials.

INTRODUCTION

Once considered one of the most treatment-refractory malignancies, melanoma is now amenable to treatment with effective systemic therapy. For the first time, new agents have been shown to improve overall survival (OS) for patients with unresectable metastatic melanoma in randomized phase III clinical trials.[1] Despite these advances, most patients who develop recurrent melanoma after seemingly curative surgery eventually die of the disease. Adjuvant interferon (IFN) therapy—the use of a year or more of IFN treatment after surgery to eradicate micrometastatic residual disease—has been shown repeatedly to delay recurrence in patients with high-risk melanoma, and probably cures a few patients, but at the expense of substantial toxicity.[2–4] Ongoing clinical

Financial Disclosures: Dr V.K. Sondak is a compensated consultant for Bristol-Myers Squibb, GlaxoSmithKline, Merck, Navidea, Novartis and Provectus. Dr G.T. Gibney is a compensated consultant for Genentech-Roche.
[a] Department of Cutaneous Oncology, Moffitt Cancer Center, 12902 Magnolia Drive, Tampa, FL 33612, USA; [b] Department of Oncologic Sciences, USF Morsani College of Medicine, 12901 Bruce B. Downs Boulevard, Tampa, FL 33612, USA
* Corresponding author. Department of Cutaneous Oncology, Moffitt Cancer Center, 12902 Magnolia Drive, Tampa, FL 33612.
E-mail address: vernon.sondak@moffitt.org

trials are testing new immunologic and molecularly targeted agents to see whether they might offer improvements over IFN when used in the adjuvant setting. Surgeons must be aware of the latest indications for systemic therapy of melanoma to make the best treatment choices and recommendations for their patients.

RELEVANT BIOLOGY BEHIND CURRENT AND NEW MELANOMA TREATMENTS
Immunotherapy

Vaccines contain tumor-associated antigens and aim to provoke an antigen-specific immune response, generally with minimal toxicity. Although they have been extensively tested in patients with melanoma, none has yet shown significant benefits in the prevention or treatment of melanoma.[5,6] However, vaccines may have their best chance for success in the prevention of metastasis; that is, in the adjuvant setting after surgery.[7] Interferon and interleukin-2 (IL-2) are powerful immunostimulating drugs that have multiple but nonspecific effects and cause significant toxicity. Interleukin-2 has never been fully evaluated in the adjuvant setting but is approved for use in treating unresectable metastatic melanoma. When used as a single agent in carefully selected patients, it is given in high doses requiring inpatient hospitalization and sometimes intensive care unit support, and is associated with a low response rate. However, some of those responses are durable and may even represent cures of patients with unresectable metastatic disease.[8] Currently, IL-2 is being investigated in conjunction with adoptive cell therapy, specifically with autologous tumor-infiltrating lymphocytes (TIL) harvested from an excised tumor and then grown ex vivo in the laboratory for patients with metastatic melanoma.[9,10] The potential advantage of this approach is a higher response rate for treated patients, with the hope that it will increase the number of patients who can experience long-term disease control and cure. In contrast to IL-2, IFN has never been widely used for metastatic disease but has been extensively tested and used clinically in the adjuvant setting for patients at high risk of recurrence after surgery.

Newer immunotherapy agents have been developed based on an improved understanding of how the antitumor immune response is regulated. Regulatory proteins on the surface of T cells can be targeted with monoclonal antibodies, resulting in the restoration of immunity for T cells that are suppressed or exhausted.[11] Ipilimumab is an antibody against CTLA-4, a negative regulatory checkpoint protein that is expressed on the surface of T cells. In patients with unresectable metastatic melanoma, one study showed that 4 doses of ipilimumab given intravenously every 3 weeks improved OS compared with a peptide vaccine, at the expense of significant immune-related adverse events in a percentage of patients.[12] These adverse events are generally manageable with steroids or other immunosuppressive drugs,[13] and ipilimumab has become a standard approach in the treatment of these patients. Given its value in metastatic disease, ipilimumab has now been used in several adjuvant therapy trials, either compared with placebo or IFN. Mature results from these trials are eagerly awaited.

Other checkpoint proteins have now been identified, and antibodies against several are in clinical trials in metastatic melanoma and other tumor types. Furthest along in clinical testing are antibodies against PD-1, a checkpoint protein expressed on exhausted T cells.[14] Anti–PD-1 antibodies, such as nivolumab and pembrolizumab (formerly called lambrolizumab or MK-3475), are being tested alone[15,16] and in combination with ipilimumab,[17] and early-phase trials suggest that anti–PD-1 antibodies may have higher response and lower toxicity rates than ipilimumab, as well as improved OS compared to chemotherapy. Because PD-1 on T cells binds to its ligand PD-L1 on the surface of tumor cells, PD-L1 expression on tumor could be a biomarker of responsiveness to anti–PD-1 antibody therapy.[18] However, at least some patients whose tumors lack PD-L1 expression have still experienced response to anti–PD-1 treatment.[19] The toxicity profile of anti–PD-1 antibodies certainly suggests that these agents could be ideal to test in adjuvant therapy trials, and these trials are just beginning to occur.

Molecularly Targeted Therapies

The discovery that about half of all cutaneous melanomas harbor mutations in the *BRAF* gene led rapidly to the development of drugs that inhibit the BRAF protein.[20] Vemurafenib and dabrafenib are 2 such drugs, and both are orally administered and lead to dramatic shrinkage of tumors in a very high percentage of patients whose tumors have the *BRAF* V600E mutation, which is by far the most common type of *BRAF* mutation.[21,22] Most responses, however, are short-lived, and resistance to treatment eventually emerges in most melanomas. In addition, treatment with BRAF inhibitors can lead to the induction of second primary cancers, including squamous cell carcinomas of the skin and new primary *BRAF* wild-type melanomas.[23,24] Immediately downstream of BRAF in the mitogen-activated protein (MAP) kinase pathway is the protein MEK, and MEK inhibitors such as trametinib also can cause responses in patients with *BRAF* mutations and some other melanomas with MAP kinase pathway activation.[25] However, the greatest value of MEK inhibitors to date has been in combination with BRAF inhibitors: studies of dabrafenib and trametinib given together indicate the combination has higher response rates, longer response duration, and less induction of secondary squamous cell carcinomas than dabrafenib alone.[26]

AN ALGORITHM FOR TREATING STAGE IV MELANOMA

The introduction of new immunologic and molecularly targeted therapies for patients with stage IV melanoma has led to some uncertainty about treatment selection and sequencing. In general, the algorithm presented in **Box 1** is used in the management of patients with newly diagnosed stage IV melanoma.[27] Patients, especially those with only one or a few metastatic deposits, are first evaluated for possible resection of all metastatic disease. If resection can render a patient completely disease-free, at least to the limits of modern imaging technology, with acceptable morbidity, this is the authors' preferred first treatment option, because a single operation can lead to long-term disease control in a small but significant number of patients.[28,29] Most patients will experience disease relapse after surgery, some quickly, and therefore the authors always consider enrolling patients with stage IV resected melanoma into a clinical trial of adjuvant therapy if available and appropriate. In one study of patients who developed stage IV melanoma after initially being enrolled onto the Multicenter Selective Lymphadenectomy Trial 1 evaluating sentinel node biopsy, an astonishing 55% were able to undergo surgery as a component of their initial treatment of stage IV melanoma.[29] This high percentage likely reflects the selection criteria that were part of the original clinical trial, because in unselected series of patients with stage IV melanoma, the number who are initially resectable is much lower ($\leq$10%).[30]

For patients who are deemed unresectable or develop unresectable recurrences after initial surgical management, the authors evaluate suitability for IL-2 therapy, either as single-agent treatment or as part of a clinical trial involving IL-2 plus adoptive cell therapy with autologous TIL. Only younger patients with no major comorbidities are considered candidates for IL-2, and consideration is usually further restricted to only those with asymptomatic disease and low total tumor burden. For adoptive cell therapy trials, the patient must also have at least one tumor nodule greater than

---

Box 1
Example algorithm for the management of patients with newly diagnosed stage IV melanoma

1. Evaluate for resectability of all identifiable disease

   a. If resectable to no evidence of disease (NED) state with acceptable morbidity/mortality: resect

   b. If not resectable to NED state with acceptable morbidity/mortality: evaluate for IL-2/TIL

2. Evaluate for candidacy for IL-2/TIL therapy

   a. Asymptomatic metastases, low tumor burden/normal lactate dehydrogenase, no or very few comorbidities: candidate for IL-2, consider for TIL trial

      i. Trial of TIL therapy available, tumor available for harvest with low morbidity: refer for TIL trial

      ii. Trial of TIL therapy not available or no suitable tumor available for harvest: consider for IL-2

   b. All other patients and patients with progressive disease despite surgery and/or IL-2/TIL: test tumor for *BRAF* with or without *KIT* mutation status and evaluate for ipilimumab

3. *BRAF* wild-type, no *KIT* mutation: consider for ipilimumab

4. *BRAF* V600E[a]:

   a. Asymptomatic metastases, low tumor burden, good performance status: consider for ipilimumab

   b. Symptomatic metastases, high tumor burden, poor performance status: initiate BRAF inhibitor with or without MEK inhibitor therapy

5. *KIT* mutation:

   a. Asymptomatic metastases, low tumor burden, good performance status: consider for ipilimumab

   b. Symptomatic metastases, high tumor burden, poor performance status: consider for KIT inhibitor therapy

Note: Always consider patients for clinical trials when available.

[a] Some other *BRAF* mutations may also respond to BRAF inhibitor therapy. See Kaufman et al[27] and clinical practice guidelines such as the NCCN Clinical Practice Guidelines in Oncology for Melanoma[51] for further details.

---

1 cm in diameter that is superficial or otherwise readily accessible for excision as a source of autologous TIL. Although only a few patients will be candidates for IL-2 treatment and the overall response rate is low, some patients have very durable responses after just a few months of treatment. Moreover, the authors prefer to treat patients with IL-2 before the administration of other immunotherapies, such as ipilimumab, which may induce toxicities that make the patient a poor candidate for IL-2 (whereas the converse situation of IL-2 treatment making a patient ineligible for ipilimumab is much less likely to occur).

BRAF-Mutant or Wild-Type Melanoma

Most patients presenting with stage IV melanoma are not candidates for either surgery or IL-2, and for these patients the decision making about therapy begins (but does not end) with knowing the *BRAF* mutation status. A representative tumor sample from paraffin-embedded formalin-fixed tissue is analyzed using one of several commercially available tests to determine the presence or absence of a treatable mutation.[31] Occasionally heterogeneity in mutation status exists between the primary and metastatic sites, or even between metastases from 2 different sites,[32] but in general the results correlate across all sites, and therefore the choice of which tumor to test is not usually a critical one. However, knowing the mutation status is just the beginning: it allows potential options to be identified, but does not bind treatment to molecularly targeted therapeutic strategies in all cases wherein the mutation is found.

In fact, many patients whose tumors are found to contain a *BRAF* gene mutation are first treated with immunotherapy, as are most patients who are found to lack a treatable *BRAF* mutation. Two main reasons exist for this: (1) although response rates are generally lower for immunotherapy than for molecularly targeted drugs, the immunotherapy responses that do occur tend to be much longer lasting than the typical response to targeted agents, and (2) salvage therapy with molecularly targeted drugs after failure of immunotherapy seems to be more effective than the other way around. As new combinations are tested and understanding of the molecular causes of resistance increases, it is likely that practitioners will be better able to choose which patients with *BRAF*-mutant melanoma should be treated first with which therapeutic approach, but for now, most patients with asymptomatic metastases and lower tumor burden are selected for immunotherapy. Patients with symptomatic metastases, a high tumor burden or rapidly progressing tumors are currently treated with molecularly targeted therapy if a *BRAF* mutation was found. Increasingly, the first-line approach to molecularly targeted therapy is combination treatment with both a BRAF and a MEK inhibitor; dabrafenib and trametinib are the first combination treatment of any kind approved by the US Food and Drug Administration (FDA) for unresectable metastatic melanoma. Several large randomized trials are testing various different BRAF/MEK inhibitor combinations and comparing them with single-agent therapy, and therefore more high-level evidence about the best first-line molecularly targeted treatment strategy will likely be available in the near future. Also under active investigation are molecularly targeted approaches for patients whose melanoma contains other less common mutations, such as those in the *NRAS* and *KIT* genes.[33]

At whatever point the patient's disease is on the treatment algorithm, and especially when indicated treatments fail, enrollment in a clinical trial should always be considered. Furthermore, at initial diagnosis of stage IV melanoma and each time treatment failure becomes evident, patients should be restaged, with particular emphasis on identifying the presence of brain metastases. In the past, the presence of brain metastases was considered to be an exclusion criterion for most clinical trials, but the widespread availability of stereotactic radiation has changed the outlook for patients with central nervous system involvement.[34] Finally, chemotherapy still has a role to play in patients who have exhausted other options. Dacarbazine chemotherapy and the closely related oral drug temozolomide are frequently used as single agents but have low response rates, and the responses that do occur are generally of short duration.[35] Nab-paclitaxel, a drug widely used in some other forms of metastatic cancer, conferred superior progression-free survival compared with dacarbazine in a phase III trial,[36] but as yet has not received FDA approval for use in patients with melanoma. The combination of carboplatin and paclitaxel is another commonly used chemotherapy regimen that has shown activity in metastatic melanoma,[37] but has never been formally compared head-to-head with dacarbazine or the component agents alone.

ADJUVANT THERAPY OF HIGH-RISK MELANOMA
Definition of High-Risk Melanoma

Most clinical trials of adjuvant therapy have focused on node-positive (stage III) melanoma, and many have also included thick, node-negative (T4a/b,N0) cases. The prognosis for patients with stage III melanoma, however, is heterogeneous, with patients with micrometastases from a nonulcerated primary (stage IIIA) having a significantly better prognosis than those in other stage III subgroups.[38] Some trials investigating more toxic regimens, such as biochemotherapy and ipilimumab, have excluded some or all patients with stage IIIA disease and focused on the higher-risk subgroups of node-positive cases. Patients with resected stage IV melanoma are at very high risk of recurrence and have increasingly been included in adjuvant therapy trials.[39] Although patients with intermediate-thickness node-negative melanoma (T2–3,N0) are not considered to be at high risk of recurrence, the large number of patients in this category means that a substantial number of melanoma-related deaths occur among these patients, especially when the primary melanoma is ulcerated.[40] Therefore, they are certainly appropriate candidates for clinical trials investigating less toxic regimens.

Results of Adjuvant Therapy with Interferon

High-dose IFN is a 1 year adjuvant therapy regimen involving 2 components: a 1-month induction phase in which 20 million units of IFN per square meter of body surface area are administered intravenously 5 days per week for 4 weeks, followed by an 11-month maintenance phase in which 10 million units per square meter of body surface area are administered subcutaneously 3 times a week.[41] The relative importance of each phase has not been adequately defined, but the 4-week induction phase alone does seem to be inadequate.[42] Three randomized trials have shown that high-dose IFN is associated with improved relapse-free survival (RFS) (delayed recurrence), and 2 trials have also shown improved OS.[2,41] In the United States, high-dose IFN is approved for use in the adjuvant therapy of thick, node-negative and node-positive melanoma. To date, no studies of high-dose IFN have defined subsets of patients who clearly respond better or worse to treatment.

Adjuvant IFN regimens involving lower doses (3–10 million units administered 3 times a week not adjusted for body surface area and without the initial intravenous component) have also been tested, but in most cases not compared directly with high-dose IFN.[2,43,44] Low-dose IFN is approved for adjuvant use in some European countries, and also has been advocated for use in intermediate-thickness, node-negative melanoma.[45] In the absence of direct comparisons between high- and low-dose IFN regimens, meta-analyses have been performed to assess the overall and comparative efficacy of adjuvant IFN therapy.[3,4] Meta-analysis results clearly support that IFN therapy delays recurrence, with an overall RFS improvement of 17% in the latest aggregated analysis,[4] but do not identify clear differences between high- and low-dose regimens in efficacy. Meta-analysis results also show a statistically significant improvement in OS for adjuvant IFN (9%). To put this improvement in context, for patients with a 40% risk of death from melanoma (as might be expected for those with stage IIIA melanoma), treating 100 of these patients with adjuvant IFN would be expected to cure 3 or 4. However, this magnitude of improvement is not dissimilar to that seen with widely accepted adjuvant chemotherapy regimens in other tumor types.[4,46]

Recently, pegylated IFN alpha was approved in the United States as an alternative adjuvant treatment for stage III melanoma based on the results of a single randomized trial conducted in Europe.[47] This trial showed a statistically significant improvement in RFS, consistent with trials of standard IFN, but did not show an OS benefit. However, the subset of patients with sentinel node–positive melanoma from an ulcerated primary showed a dramatic improvement in survival (41%) when treated with pegylated IFN.[47] Although some other IFN trials have shown a similar benefit in this subset,[48,49] this is best considered an unproven but provocative finding pending definitive replication. Pegylated IFN has not been directly compared with high-dose IFN but seems to have fewer serious side effects. Unlike high-dose IFN, pegylated IFN is given for up to 5 years, and the 1-month intravenously administered induction phase is replaced with a 2-month subcutaneously administered induction phase. With its longer half-life after subcutaneous injection, pegylated IFN is administered only once a week, instead of 3 times per week for standard IFN, and has pharmacologic properties that might make it a more favorable agent for the maintenance phase.[50] The treatment philosophy of the approved pegylated IFN regimen, namely that dosage should be adjusted to a level at which patients can tolerate 5 years of treatment with minimal or no impact on performance status and activities of daily life, is designed to make long-term therapy feasible and, like all IFN regimens, depends on close cooperation between the patient and treatment team for optimum results.

Clinical Trials of New Adjuvant Therapy Agents

Although the demonstrated benefits of IFN regimens justify their use in patients with high-risk melanoma who are motivated to delay or prevent recurrence, more effective adjuvant therapies are needed. The availability of new agents with documented survival benefits in unresectable metastatic melanoma has spurred trials of these agents in the adjuvant setting (**Table 1**). Whether these agents will be equally or more effective than available IFN regimens, and how the toxicities of these new drugs will be tolerated by patients who are disease-free and possibly cured at the time of treatment, remains to be seen. Nonetheless, the hope is that the advances in understanding melanoma biology and the regulators of the antitumor immune response that have

Table 1
Examples of clinical trials investigating new agents for adjuvant therapy of high-risk resected melanoma

Agent/Trial (ClinicalTrials. gov Identifier)	Disease Stage	Trial Status	Comments
Ipilimumab			
Ipilimumab, 10 mg/kg vs placebo, EORTC18071 (NCT00636168)	III	Closed to accrual	RFS significantly prolonged by ipilimumab but high rate of severe toxicity; OS data pending[52]
Ipilimumab, 10 mg/kg vs ipilimumab, 3 mg/kg vs interferon alfa, E1609 (NCT01274338)	IIIB/C, resected IVA/B	Open to accrual	Completion of accrual expected August 2014
BRAF inhibitors			
Vemurafenib vs placebo, BRIM8 (NCT01667419)	IIC or III	Open to accrual	
Dabrafenib/trametinib vs placebo, COMBI-AD (NCT01682083)	III	Open to accrual	
Anti–PD-1 antibodies			
Nivolumab ± ipilimumab plus peptide vaccine, MCC15651 (NCT01176474)	IIIC, resected IV	Open to accrual	

Abbreviations: EORTC, European Organisation for Research and Treatment of Cancer; MCC, Moffitt Cancer Center; RFS, relapse-free survival.

profoundly changed treatment for stage IV melanoma will likely eventually translate into new, more effective, and less toxic approaches to the prevention of recurrence by adjuvant therapy.

SUMMARY

Advances in the management of unresectable metastatic melanoma have significant implications for the surgical management of melanoma, and surgeons must familiarize themselves with new drugs and the biology behind them. In some cases, treatment with these new drugs can convert patients with unresectable disease into candidates for curative surgery, and clinical trials investigating the role of new agents for the prevention of recurrence are likely to transform melanoma care in the future, just as they have for patients with widespread metastatic disease.

REFERENCES

1. McArthur GA, Ribas A. Targeting oncogenic drivers and the immune system in melanoma. J Clin Oncol 2013;31:499–506.
2. Kirkwood JM, Manola J, Ibrahim J, et al. A pooled analysis of Eastern Cooperative Oncology Group and intergroup trials of adjuvant high-dose interferon for melanoma. Clin Cancer Res 2004;10:1670–7.
3. Mocellin S, Pasquali S, Rossi CR, et al. Interferon alpha adjuvant therapy in patients with high-risk melanoma: a systematic review and meta-analysis. J Natl Cancer Inst 2010;102:493–501.
4. Mocellin S, Lens MB, Pasquali S, et al. Interferon alpha for the adjuvant treatment of cutaneous melanoma. Cochrane Database Syst Rev 2013;(6):CD008955.
5. Sondak VK, Liu PY, Tuthill RJ, et al. Adjuvant immunotherapy of resected, intermediate-thickness node-negative melanoma with an allogeneic tumor vaccine. Overall results of a randomized trial of the Southwest Oncology Group. J Clin Oncol 2002;20:2058–66.
6. Rosenberg SA, Yang JC, Restifo NP. Cancer immunotherapy: moving beyond current vaccines. Nat Med 2004;10:909–15.
7. Sosman JA, Weeraratna AT, Sondak VK. When will melanoma vaccines be proven effective? J Clin Oncol 2004;22:387–9.
8. Schwartzentruber DJ, Lawson DH, Richards JM, et al. gp100 peptide vaccine and interleukin-2 in patients with advanced melanoma. N Engl J Med 2011; 364:2119–27.
9. Rosenberg SA, Yang JC, Sherry RM, et al. Durable complete responses in heavily pretreated patients with metastatic melanoma using T-cell transfer immunotherapy. Clin Cancer Res 2011;17:4550–7.
10. Pilon-Thomas S, Kuhn L, Ellwanger S, et al. Efficacy of adoptive cell transfer of tumor-infiltrating lymphocytes after lymphopenia induction for metastatic melanoma. J Immunother 2012;35:615–20.
11. Yao S, Zhu Y, Chen L. Advances in targeting cell surface signalling molecules for immune modulation. Nat Rev Drug Discov 2013;12:130–46.
12. Hodi FS, O'Day SJ, McDermott DF, et al. Improved survival with ipilimumab in patients with metastatic melanoma. N Engl J Med 2010;363:711–23.
13. Phan GQ, Weber JS, Sondak VK. CTLA-4 blockade with monoclonal antibodies in patients with metastatic cancer: surgical issues. Ann Surg Oncol 2008;15:3014–21.
14. Ott PA, Hodi FS, Robert C. CTLA-4 and PD-1/PD-L1 blockade: new immunotherapeutic modalities with durable clinical benefit in melanoma patients. Clin Cancer Res 2013;19:5300–9.

15. Topalian SL, Sznol M, McDermott DF, et al. Survival, durable tumor remission, and long-term safety in patients with advanced melanoma receiving nivolumab. J Clin Oncol 2014;32:1020–30.
16. Hamid O, Robert C, Daud A, et al. Safety and tumor responses with lambrolizumab (anti-PD-1) in melanoma. N Engl J Med 2013;369:134–44.
17. Wolchok JD, Kluger H, Callahan MK, et al. Nivolumab plus ipilimumab in advanced melanoma. N Engl J Med 2013;369:122–33.
18. Topalian SL, Hodi FS, Brahmer JR, et al. Safety, activity, and immune correlates of anti-PD-1 antibody in cancer. N Engl J Med 2012;366:2443–54.
19. Weber JS, Kudchadkar RR, Yu B, et al. Safety, efficacy, and biomarkers of nivolumab with vaccine in ipilimumab-refractory or -naive melanoma. J Clin Oncol 2013;31:4311–8.
20. Davies H, Bignell GR, Cox C, et al. Mutations of the BRAF gene in human cancer. Nature 2002;418:949–54.
21. McArthur GA, Chapman PB, Robert C, et al. Safety and efficacy of vemurafenib in BRAF(V600E) and BRAF(V600K) mutation-positive melanoma (BRIM-3): extended follow-up of a phase 3, randomised, open-label study. Lancet Oncol 2014;15:323–32.
22. Hauschild A, Grob JJ, Demidov LV, et al. Dabrafenib in BRAF-mutated metastatic melanoma: a multicentre, open-label, phase 3 randomised controlled trial. Lancet 2012;380:358–65.
23. Gibney GT, Messina JL, Fedorenko IV, et al. Paradoxical oncogenesis–the long-term effects of BRAF inhibition in melanoma. Nat Rev Clin Oncol 2013;10:390–9.
24. Zimmer L, Hillen U, Livingstone E, et al. Atypical melanocytic proliferations and new primary melanomas in patients with advanced melanoma undergoing selective BRAF inhibition. J Clin Oncol 2012;30:2375–83.
25. Flaherty KT, Robert C, Hersey P, et al. Improved survival with MEK inhibition in BRAF-mutated melanoma. N Engl J Med 2012;367:107–14.
26. Flaherty KT, Infante JR, Daud A, et al. Combined BRAF and MEK inhibition in melanoma with BRAF V600 mutations. N Engl J Med 2012;367:1694–703.
27. Kaufman HL, Kirkwood JK, Hodi FS, et al. The Society for Immunotherapy of Cancer consensus statement on tumour immunotherapy for the treatment of cutaneous melanoma. Nat Rev Clin Oncol 2013;10:588–98.
28. Sosman JA, Moon J, Tuthill RJ, et al. A phase 2 trial of complete resection for stage IV melanoma: results of Southwest Oncology Group clinical trial S9430. Cancer 2011;117:4740–6.
29. Howard JH, Thompson JF, Mozzillo N, et al. Metastasectomy for distant metastatic melanoma: analysis of data from the first Multicenter Selective Lymphadenectomy Trial (MSLT-I). Ann Surg Oncol 2012;19:2547–55.
30. Wevers KP, Hoekstra HJ. Stage IV melanoma: completely resectable patients are scarce. Ann Surg Oncol 2013;20:2352–6.
31. Kudchadkar R, Gibney G, Sondak VK. Integrating molecular biomarkers into current clinical management in melanoma. Methods Mol Biol 2014;1102:27–42.
32. Wilmott JS, Tembe V, Howle JR, et al. Intratumoral molecular heterogeneity in a BRAF-mutant, BRAF inhibitor-resistant melanoma: a case illustrating the challenges for personalized medicine. Mol Cancer Ther 2012;11:2704–8.
33. Hodi FS, Corless CL, Giobbie-Hurder A, et al. Imatinib for melanomas harboring mutationally activated or amplified KIT arising on mucosal, acral, and chronically sun-damaged skin. J Clin Oncol 2013;31:3182–90.
34. Kenchappa RS, Tran N, Rao NG, et al. Novel treatments for melanoma brain metastases. Cancer Control 2013;20:298–306.

35. Gibney GT, Sondak VK. Has targeted therapy for melanoma made chemotherapy obsolete? Lancet Oncol 2013;14:676–7.

36. Hersh E, Del Vecchio M, Brown M, et al. Phase 3, randomized, open-label, multicenter trial of nab-paclitaxel (nab-P) vs dacarbazine (DTIC) in previously untreated patients with metastatic malignant melanoma (MMM) [abstract]. Pigment Cell Melanoma Res 2012;25:863.

37. Flaherty KT, Lee SJ, Zhao F, et al. Phase III trial of carboplatin and paclitaxel with or without sorafenib in metastatic melanoma. J Clin Oncol 2013;31:373–9.

38. Balch CM, Gershenwald JE, Soong SJ, et al. Multivariate analysis of prognostic factors among 2,313 patients with stage III melanoma: comparison of nodal micrometastases versus macrometastases. J Clin Oncol 2010;28:2452–9.

39. Sarnaik AA, Yu B, Yu D, et al. Extended dose ipilimumab with a peptide vaccine: immune correlates associated with clinical benefit in patients with resected high-risk stage IIIc/IV melanoma. Clin Cancer Res 2011;17:896–906.

40. Morton DL, Thompson JF, Cochran AJ, et al. Sentinel-node biopsy or nodal observation in melanoma. N Engl J Med 2006;355:1307–17.

41. Kirkwood JM, Strawderman MH, Ernstoff MS, et al. Interferon alfa-2b adjuvant therapy of high-risk resected cutaneous melanoma: the Eastern Cooperative Oncology Group Trial EST 1684. J Clin Oncol 1996;14:7–17.

42. McArthur GA. Adjuvant interferon in melanoma: is duration of therapy important? J Clin Oncol 2014;32:171–3.

43. Hancock BW, Wheatley K, Harris S, et al. Adjuvant interferon in high-risk melanoma: the AIM HIGH Study–United Kingdom Coordinating Committee on Cancer Research randomized study of adjuvant low-dose extended-duration interferon alfa-2a in high-risk resected malignant melanoma. J Clin Oncol 2004;22:53–61.

44. Schuchter LM. Adjuvant interferon therapy for melanoma: high-dose, low-dose, no dose, which dose? J Clin Oncol 2004;22:7–10.

45. Grob JJ, Dreno B, de la Salmonière P, et al. Randomised trial of interferon alpha-2a as adjuvant therapy in resected primary melanoma thicker than 1.5 mm without clinically detectable node metastases. Lancet 1998;351:1905–10.

46. Ascierto PA, Kirkwood JM. Adjuvant therapy of melanoma with interferon: lessons of the past decade. J Transl Med 2008;6:62.

47. Eggermont AM, Suciu S, Testori A, et al. Long-term results of the randomized phase III trial EORTC 18991 of adjuvant therapy with pegylated interferon alfa-2b versus observation in resected stage III melanoma. J Clin Oncol 2012;30:3810–8.

48. McMasters KM, Edwards MJ, Ross MI, et al. Ulceration as a predictive marker for response to adjuvant interferon therapy in melanoma. Ann Surg 2010;252:460–5.

49. Eggermont AM, Suciu S, Testori A, et al. Ulceration and stage are predictive of interferon efficacy in melanoma: results of the phase III adjuvant trials EORTC 18952 and EORTC 18991. Eur J Cancer 2012;48:218–25.

50. Daud AI, Xu C, Hwu WJ, et al. Pharmacokinetic/pharmacodynamic analysis of adjuvant pegylated interferon α-2b in patients with resected high-risk melanoma. Cancer Chemother Pharmacol 2011;67:657–66.

51. Coit DG, Thompson JA, Andtbacka R, et al. NCCN Clinical Practice Guidelines in Oncology: Melanoma. Version 4, 2014. Available at: NCCN.org. Accessed July 19, 2014.

52. Eggermont AM, Chiarion-Sileni V, Grob JJ, et al. Ipilimumab versus placebo after complete resection of stage III melanoma: initial efficacy and safety results from the EORTC 18071 phase III trial. J Clin Oncol 2014;32(Suppl):LBA9008.

Unusual Presentations of Melanoma

Melanoma of Unknown Primary Site, Melanoma Arising in Childhood, and Melanoma Arising in the Eye and on Mucosal Surfaces

Vernon K. Sondak, MD[a,b,c,*], Jane L. Messina, MD[a,d,e,f]

KEYWORDS

- Melanoma • Unknown primary • Pediatric melanoma • Mucosal melanoma
- Uveal melanoma • Immunotherapy • Targeted therapy • Adjuvant therapy

KEY POINTS

- Major advances have occurred in our understanding of cutaneous melanoma in adults, but these have not yet translated into significant breakthroughs for the management of melanomas arising in noncutaneous locations such as the eye and mucosal surfaces.
- Management of melanoma arising in children remains controversial.
- Melanoma presenting in regional lymph nodes without a known cutaneous primary site behaves in a manner entirely consistent with recurrence after removal of a known primary, and should therefore be managed in an analogous fashion.
- New molecular tests, including gene expression profiling and comparative genomic hybridization, have been introduced for evaluation of uveal and pediatric melanomas, but their optimal role in patient management remains to be defined.

Financial Disclosures: Dr V.K. Sondak is a compensated consultant for Bristol-Myers Squibb, GlaxoSmithKline, Merck, Navidea, Novartis and Provectus.
[a] Department of Cutaneous Oncology, Moffitt Cancer Center, 12902 Magnolia Drive, Tampa, FL 33612, USA; [b] Department of Oncologic Sciences, USF Morsani College of Medicine, 12901 Bruce B. Downs Boulevard, Tampa, FL 33612, USA; [c] Department of Surgery, USF Morsani College of Medicine, 12901 Bruce B. Downs Boulevard, Tampa, FL 33612, USA; [d] Department of Anatomic Pathology, Moffitt Cancer Center, 12902 Magnolia Drive, Tampa, FL 33612, USA; [e] Department of Pathology & Cell Biology, USF Morsani College of Medicine, 12901 Bruce B. Downs Boulevard, Tampa, FL 33612, USA; [f] Department of Dermatology, USF Morsani College of Medicine, 12901 Bruce B. Downs Boulevard, Tampa, FL 33612, USA
* Corresponding author. Department of Cutaneous Oncology, Moffitt Cancer Center, 12902 Magnolia Drive, Tampa, FL 33612.
E-mail address: vernon.sondak@moffitt.org

INTRODUCTION

More than 90% of all melanomas present as primary tumors on the skin surface, and most are diagnosed during adulthood. About 5% of all melanomas arise in the eye, and 1% to 2% arise on the mucosal surfaces or present as apparently metastatic disease somewhere other than on the skin without any known history of a cutaneous primary melanoma.[1] Melanoma is being diagnosed in pediatric age patients more frequently than ever before.[2] Surgeons need to be aware of these unusual presentations of melanoma, and in particular to understand the important site-specific differences in biology and management compared with the 'typical' adult patient presenting with a cutaneous primary melanoma.

UNKNOWN PRIMARY MELANOMA IN REGIONAL NODES

A review of the National Cancer Data Base found that 2.2% of all melanoma patients presented without a known primary site.[1] The same review found that 23.1% of cutaneous melanoma patients presented with stage III disease (nodal or intralymphatic involvement). Among melanoma patients presenting with palpable lymph nodes, however, between 13% and 17% have no known primary site.[3,4] Potential explanations for this unusual presentation include removal of the original primary on the skin without recognizing it as malignant (eg, cryoablation of a presumed nonmelanoma skin cancer, misdiagnosis of a biopsy specimen as a benign nevus, unrecognized accidental or traumatic amputation of the primary), regression of the original primary with persistence of a clone of metastatic cells in the regional node, and primary malignant degeneration of intranodal melanocytes (nodal nevus cells). However, it is not unusual for a careful physical examination to turn up an occult primary site in a patient referred in with "an unknown primary."

Initial Evaluation

Initial evaluation of the patient includes evaluating these various potential explanations, as well as the typical evaluation of the stage III melanoma patient for resectability and the possibility of occult distant metastatic disease. A thorough history includes detailed questioning about traumatized, regressed, ablated, or removed pigmented or amelanotic lesions located anywhere in the draining field of the involved nodal basin. For the inguinal nodes, the questioning should also encompass any history of hemorrhoids and lesions on the genitalia, as well as on the toes and soles of the feet. If the patient relates a history of a benign nevus having been removed from the relevant anatomic region, efforts to secure the pathology report and/or the slides for secondary review can be helpful. If the patient relates a history of a regressed pigmented skin lesion, they may have old photographs that document the lesion's original appearance. Physical examination should follow up on any areas identified during the history, and look for unrecognized pigmented or amelanotic lesions and unexplained scars or hypopigmented areas. The physical can be supplemented by examination using a Wood's lamp ("black light") to highlight areas of hypopigmentation for further evaluation. Direct ophthalmoscopy can be carried out, but the likelihood that a nodal metastasis is arising from a uveal primary site is extremely remote, and routine referral to an ophthalmologist is not required in the absence of visual symptoms or suspected abnormalities seen on ophthalmoscopy. For inguinal lymphadenopathy, rectal and (for females) pelvic examinations are appropriate, with more detailed evaluation or referral for gynecologic examination or endoscopy if findings warrant. For cervical lymphadenopathy, the possibility of a nasal or oropharyngeal mucosal primary should be entertained, and referral for endoscopy considered.

The staging workup is similar to that for palpable stage III melanoma from a known primary, and includes cross-sectional imaging (whole body positron emission tomography (PET)/computed tomography (CT) or CT of the chest and abdomen, with inclusion of the pelvis or neck depending on the site of nodal disease) and evaluation of the central nervous system (contrast-enhanced brain magnetic resonance imaging, with CT if magnetic resonance imaging is contraindicated or the patient is severely claustrophobic). We often add ultrasound evaluation of other nodal basins, particularly if we suspect that the original primary lesion might have arisen on an area of skin with ambiguous lymphatic drainage.

Relevant Biology

Emerging data suggest that the mutational status of unknown primary melanomas within the regional nodes closely mirrors the pattern seen with known cutaneous primaries, with approximately half of cases harboring *BRAF* V600 mutations.[5] This finding lends support to the notion that most, if not all, cases of nodal unknown primary melanoma represent metastases from an original cutaneous primary. Overall, the outcome for patients with unknown primary melanomas within the regional nodes is slightly better than that for all patients with macroscopic stage III melanoma from a known primary site. In one series, the 5-year survival rates were 55% for patients with an unknown primary compared with 42% for those with a known primary ($P = .04$),[3] whereas in another the rates were 55% versus 44% ($P = .002$).[4] This has led to speculation that an antitumor immune response led to regression of the primary site and potentially a favorable systemic response as well. However, available evidence suggests that in fact the prognosis for unknown primary patients is identical to known primary patients presenting with metachronous nodal metastasis, and that both groups have a more favorable survival than patients presenting with synchronous nodal metastasis at the time of diagnosis of the primary cutaneous melanoma.[6,7] Moreover, in our experience with cases where a previous lesion has been biopsied on the skin and misdiagnosed as benign, subsequent pathology re-review generally has shown the lesion to be a relatively thin melanoma with nevus-like features and few or absent mitoses. If so, it would not be surprising that, when such lesions eventually metastasize, the outcome might be slightly more favorable than average.

Surgical Management

Overall, we believe the prognosis of unknown primary melanoma presenting in the lymph nodes is identical to that for patients with known cutaneous primaries and metachronous lymph node metastases, and hence the surgical management is almost exactly the same, namely, radical lymphadenectomy. We are slightly less inclined to perform a pelvic lymphadenectomy for unknown primary patients presenting with inguinal nodal involvement and radiographically negative pelvic nodes than would be the case for known primary patients, because of the possibility that the original primary might have lymphatic drainage to both groins or to the groin and the axilla. If the preoperative evaluation uncovered any areas of hypopigmentation or other suspect skin lesions, these are removed at the time of radical lymphadenectomy for histopathologic evaluation.

Adjuvant Therapy

Postoperatively, identical criteria are used for decision making about adjuvant systemic therapy and adjuvant radiation as would be employed for patients with a known cutaneous primary. Adjuvant interferon (IFN) alfa-2b has been repeatedly shown in multiple clinical trials to improve relapse-free survival[8,9] and, in metaanalyses, to have a small but statistically significant impact on overall survival.[10] Its use should be considered in appropriately selected patients. Most important, patients with unknown primary melanoma in regional nodes should be considered appropriate candidates for participation in clinical trials testing new forms of adjuvant therapy, and not excluded from these trials because of an anticipated difference in prognosis and natural history from other types of stage III melanoma patients. Examples of recent adjuvant therapy trials that successfully included unknown primary stage III melanoma patients are the Southwest Oncology Group trial S0008 (NCT00006237) and the Eastern Cooperative Oncology Group trial E1609 (NCT01274338), which compare high-dose IFN with bio-chemotherapy and ipilimumab (anti-CTLA4 antibody), respectively.

Adjuvant radiation to the regional nodal basin has been shown in a randomized trial to significantly decrease the likelihood of in-field relapse, but not improve relapse-free survival or overall survival, in high-risk patients after radical lymphadenectomy.[11] Many patients who present with stage III melanoma from an unknown primary meet the study's criteria for high-risk disease: Extranodal extension of tumor present, mul-tiple (≥ 1 parotid, ≥ 2 cervical or axillary, or ≥ 3 inguinal) tumor-containing nodes, or maximum size of any one involved node >3 cm for a cervical node or >4 cm for an axil-lary or inguinal node. Indeed, 18.1% of patients in this trial had an unknown primary site. For all patients in this study, the risk of lymph node basin relapse was reduced from 20.6% to 6.6%,[11] but at the expense of increased short- and long-term toxicity. What remains unknown at this time is whether and how often patients who suffered lymph node basin relapse on the control arm could be salvaged by re-resection, radi-ation, or both, restricting the morbidity of nodal basin irradiation only to those who actually recurred regionally. Until more data become available, decision making about adjuvant radiation should be personalized to reflect the risk of an in-basin relapse, the salvage options available and the relative risk of long-term complications from radi-ating that nodal basin (eg, there is a greater risk of lymphedema from radiating inguinal than axillary nodes).

Some patients with unknown primary melanoma in the lymph nodes present at a very advanced stage, with the resectability of the disease either questionable or un-equivocally not feasible without unacceptable morbidity. In those cases, neoadjuvant therapy should be strongly considered based on *BRAF* mutation status: Patients with *BRAF* V600 mutations are potentially good candidates for neoadjuvant targeted ther-apy with BRAF plus or minus MEK inhibitors. The objective response rate to targeted therapy in unresectable stage III disease is >50%,[12,13] and possibly as high as 75% to 80% for combination therapy,[14] so many patients would be expected to be converted to a clearly resectable state after only a few months of treatment. Although the situa-tion is not quite as favorable for patients lacking a targetable *BRAF* mutation, recent trials of anti-PD1 antibodies alone[15] or with ipilimumab[16] have shown response rates nearly as high and hence hold promise to offer another form of neoadjuvant therapy for converting borderline resectable or unresectable disease to a resectable state.

UNKNOWN PRIMARY MELANOMA IN THE DERMIS AND SUBCUTANEOUS TISSUE

Not infrequently, although the precise incidence is poorly defined, patients present with a single dermal or subcutaneous nodule of melanoma and the pathologist is un-able to identify an epidermal component to establish the diagnosis of primary cuta-neous melanoma.[17] The American Joint Committee on Cancer staging guidelines for melanoma indicate that, "when there are localized metastases to the skin or sub-cutaneous tissues, these should... be presumed to be regional (ie, stage III instead of stage IV) if an appropriate staging workup does not reveal any other sites of metastases."[18] However, the basis for considering such a lesion to represent stage III disease is unclear. In fact, available evidence suggests that these dermal or subcutaneous tumors are usually primary melanomas where the epidermal component has regressed or been lost, such as by prior biopsy, trauma (such as repeated scratching), or cryoablation. Traumatic removal of the epidermal component of a melanoma is not infrequent in areas groomed by shaving, such as the legs in women and face in men. For tumors centered in the deep dermis or subcutaneous tissue, a diagnosis of clear cell sarcoma should be entertained, and the specimen referred for analysis for the t(12;22)(q13;q12) translocation when appropriate.

Melanomas located in the dermis and subcutaneous tissue behave more like thick primary melanomas or local recurrences than regional metastases, and it is generally our practice to treat them as such. In at least some cases, this type of melanoma may have arisen as a primary tumor within the dermis ("primary dermal melanoma"), and hence does not represent a truly unknown primary.[17,19] Management of these cases benefits greatly from close collaboration with the pathologist as well as a careful history to seek evidence for an initial cutaneous component of the tumor versus a history of a primary melanoma at another site that could have potentially been the source of metastasis. A full metastatic workup may or may not be ordered depending on the level of uncertainty about the possibility that the lesion might represent a primary tumor and the size of the nodule itself, and regional nodal ultrasonography is frequently employed as well. Most cases are managed as if they were a known cutaneous melanoma of equal thickness, that is, by wide excision and sentinel lymph node biopsy, if not otherwise contraindicated. Not infrequently, the presence of an epidermal component is noted in the wide excision specimen, in retrospect establishing these lesions as primary cutaneous melanoma after all.

UNKNOWN PRIMARY MELANOMA IN VISCERAL ORGANS

The most challenging scenarios are presented by cases of melanoma developing in visceral sites without a known cutaneous primary. All of the considerations regarding a regressed, traumatized, or misdiagnosed primary tumor mentioned for stage III unknown primary must be considered when evaluating a case of presumed stage IV unknown primary melanoma. Just as the location of the nodal disease can point toward possible primary sites in stage III unknown primary cases, the pattern of metastatic disease can point toward possible primary sites in stage IV cases. For example, because uveal melanoma metastasizes so frequently to the liver, when a patient presents with widespread metastatic melanoma in the liver without a known primary, an appropriate ophthalmologic evaluation should be undertaken. When the visceral melanoma is found in a single site, such as the gastrointestinal tract, the possibility of a visceral primary rather than metastatic disease from an unknown primary must be entertained seriously. Recently, genetic characterization of tumors felt to represent unknown primary metastatic melanoma in the small intestine and other sites have revealed some of these tumors to have the characteristic chromosomal translocation of clear cell sarcoma,[20] suggesting that they were in fact primary sarcomas and not melanoma metastases. Currently, when faced with a patient with an isolated lesion consistent with metastatic melanoma but no known cutaneous or ocular primary site, we use standard molecular testing for *BRAF* mutations and also send the tumor for analysis for the t(12;22)(q13;q12) translocation, resulting in the fusion protein EWSR1/ATF1, to evaluate for the possibility the tumor is actually a primary clear cell sarcoma. At present, however, the management is the same whether or not the translocation is found: A full metastatic workup including cross-sectional body and brain imaging, with resection of an isolated lesion whenever possible. Unlike stage III melanoma of unknown primary origin, the role of adjuvant therapy is less clear for stage IV unknown primary melanoma (and completely unknown for primary clear cell sarcoma of the gastrointestinal tract). Overall, however, the outcome for patients with unknown primary stage IV melanoma seems to be more favorable than for patients with a known primary, even in matched-pair analysis compared with otherwise similar known primary cases.[21]

CUTANEOUS MELANOMA ARISING IN CHILDHOOD

Incidence rates for melanoma in children <18 years of age are rising in the United States, particularly in teenage females,[2] likely at least in part owing to the widespread use of artificial tanning.[22,23] It is also likely that increased awareness of pediatric melanoma has led more parents to seek evaluation of their children's moles and more pediatricians to biopsy or refer for biopsy those moles that they are evaluating. As a consequence, the increasing number of biopsies being performed has brought many histopathologically challenging lesions to the microscope stage, often with discordant results, even among expert dermatopathologists.[24] Hence, it is probable that the current increase in pediatric melanoma cases is a result of earlier diagnosis of some unequivocal melanomas that were previously not detected until adulthood, but also includes some cases of highly atypical melanocytic neoplasms that may have a more favorable prognosis than adult melanomas of similar thickness.[25] Together, these phenomena may explain why the prognosis for pediatric patients diagnosed with melanoma seems to be slightly more favorable than for adults.[26] However, the notion that pediatric melanoma is somehow a 'benign' disease[27] is unfortunately counteracted by numerous fatal cases even from lesions originally termed atypical rather than malignant.[24,26,28–30] Recognizing the potential number of years lost when melanoma diagnosed in the pediatric population results in death, a treatment approach similar to adult melanoma is certainly easy to justify.

Initial Evaluation

Pediatric melanomas frequently lack the characteristic ABCD properties typical of adult melanomas,[31] so a high index of suspicion is required to establish which of the many new and evolving moles of childhood should be biopsied and examined histologically. Any lesions suspected of being atypical or malignant should ideally be reviewed by a dermatopathologist with expertise in pediatric melanocytic neoplasms,[24] but the clinician must keep in mind the inevitable degree of diagnostic uncertainty with pediatric lesions. Close communication with the pathologist is always helpful. Otherwise, the initial evaluation of the patient is identical to that for a similar adult melanoma patient, albeit with the recognition that radiographic studies should be ordered with even greater awareness of the potential for adverse consequences of radiation exposure in the young.[32] The skin examination should also take note of the presence and number of typical and atypical nevi and the presence of any congenital nevi. A family history suggestive of the presence of an inherited melanoma susceptibility gene is rarely obtained, but likely accounts for a small percentage of cases.[33]

Relevant Biology

Because melanomas arising in different pediatric populations (infants, young children, older children, and teenagers or young adults) likely have different etiologic factors, it is not surprising that studies of the biology of pediatric melanoma have shown varied results. Older children with melanoma seem to have a frequency of BRAF mutation that is similar to that seen in young adults, whereas at least 1 study has shown a higher incidence of *KIT* mutation than would be anticipated in adult melanoma.[34] Molecular analysis using comparative genomic hybridization and fluorescence in situ hybridization have proven to be useful diagnostic adjuncts in discriminating benign lesions from those with poor outcome. Well-characterized findings that can assist in establishing a diagnosis include polyploidy or isolated 11p gain seen on comparative genomic hybridization in benign Spitz nevi, particularly those with a history of recurrence, as well as isolated whole chromosomal gains in proliferative nodules in congenital nevi.[35,36] Homozygous deletions of chromosome 9p21, which can result in loss of the *CDKN2A* (p16) gene, can be identified by fluorescence in situ hybridization and seem to be associated with a poorer prognosis and a greater propensity for brain metastasis.[36–38]

Operative Management

In general, pediatric melanoma seems to have a lesser risk of local recurrence and a greater incidence of nodal metastasis when compared with adult melanoma of the same thickness.[25,26,29,30,39] Accordingly, we advocate wide excision of the primary site and sentinel lymph node biopsy in keeping with standard adult guidelines, with the exception that in children younger than 14 we utilize a 1-cm margin for melanomas of all thicknesses and have not seen local recurrences with that approach.[25] The role of sentinel node biopsy in the setting of a diagnostically challenging melanocytic neoplasm is a hotly debated topic, but based on available evidence this procedure should be considered in lesions where diagnostic consensus cannot be reached after expert consultation and molecular testing, if feasible. Although the risk of nodal metastasis is higher with pediatric than adult melanoma, and is also high with pediatric atypical Spitzoid tumors, the rate of finding non–sentinel node metastases is relatively low, and the prognosis of stage III pediatric melanoma relatively better compared with adults.[26,29,30,39,40] Just as in adults with positive sentinel nodes, there is uncertainty about the exact role of completion lymph node dissection for children with sentinel node–positive melanoma and especially for those with evidence of atypical cells in the sentinel nodes from atypical Spitzoid tumors. We employ a selective policy toward completion lymphadenectomy, and when it is omitted we follow the involved nodal basin(s) with ultrasonography, just as in adult patients.

Adjuvant Therapy

IFN has been advocated for children with node-positive melanoma,[41] and pediatric patients tolerate IFN better than adults.[42,43] Although the risks of treatment must be balanced against the somewhat better prognosis for stage III melanoma in pediatric patients, these patients and their families are often highly motivated toward a proactive approach,[25] and we routinely recommend 1 year of adjuvant IFN for our node-positive pediatric melanoma patients. However, based on pharmacokinetic considerations and the desire to avoid multiple injections per week during the subcutaneously administered maintenance phase,[44] we have routinely substituted pegylated IFN[9] for standard IFN during the final 11 months of therapy. Given the potential adverse effects of radiotherapy on growth and development and morbidity, such as increased risks of lymphedema and second malignancy, we would need a very high burden of regional disease to consider adjuvant radiation in a pediatric patient and as yet have not had occasion to use it in any pediatric age melanoma patient.

MELANOMA ARISING ON MUCOSAL SURFACES

Melanocytes are found in many locations throughout the body, not just in the epidermis, so it is not unexpected that primary melanomas can arise in extracutaneous locations.

Most extracutaneous sites, however, receive little or no exposure to ultraviolet radiation, which likely explains the extremely low frequency of extracutaneous compared with cutaneous primary melanomas. Mucosal surfaces in particular likely receive no ultraviolet exposure, so the precise mechanism of melanomagenesis on these surfaces is unknown but the pattern of genetic aberrations in these tumors is quite different from those seen in melanomas arising on intermittently or chronically sun-exposed skin.[45] Melanomas arising on mucosal surfaces accounted for 1.3% to 2.0% of melanomas in large national database studies from the United States and The Netherlands, respectively.[1,46]

Site-Specific Differences

Mucosal melanomas are generally subdivided into those occurring in the head and neck (nasal, nasopharyngeal, oral, oropharyngeal, and laryngeal mucosa), gastrointestinal tract (predominantly but not exclusively anorectal mucosa), vagina, and urinary tract. It should be noted that vulvar and perianal melanomas actually arise from the cutaneous surfaces in those locations and not the mucosal surfaces, but are often lumped together with their mucosal counterparts in reports of extracutaneous melanomas. Possibly because of this, different series relate different relative frequencies of and survival rates for mucosal melanomas at the various sites, although most agree that the urinary tract mucosa is the least frequent site with among the poorest survival rates. The various mucosal sites differ in the feasibility and consequences of radical excision with wide margins, in the nature of the lymphatic drainage from the primary site and in the sensitivity of the surrounding tissues to radiation. For example, anorectal melanomas may be amenable to wide resection by means of abdominoperineal resection, whereas a nasopharyngeal melanoma might not be widely excised even with a very radical and deforming procedure. Anal, perianal, and vulvar melanomas would drain to lymph nodes in the inguinal basins and be amenable to sentinel node biopsy, whereas rectal and vaginal melanomas might also drain to pelvic nodes not easily accessible for that procedure.

Initial Evaluation

Regardless of the primary site, the initial evaluation calls for a history and physical examination elucidating symptoms or signs related to the primary tumor and evidence of regional metastasis. Symptoms are usually nonspecific, such as bleeding that is easily mistaken for hemorrhoids, nonmalignant vaginal bleeding, or epistaxis. Therefore, there is often a delay between the first symptoms and actual diagnosis. Tumors are commonly large and locally advanced, and clinically apparent nodal metastasis is not unusual at presentation. Evaluation of the primary site and regional nodes varies based on location, with endoscopy or vaginal speculum examination usually being necessary to assess the visible extent of the primary, and endorectal ultrasonography frequently required to assess for transmural penetration of the tumor, mesorectal lymphadenopathy, or both. Because locally advanced lesions are so common, a more complete staging workup to look for distant metastatic disease such as PET/CT is often justified.

Relevant Biology

Mucosal melanomas show clear genetic differences from cutaneous melanoma, in particular with fewer *BRAF* mutations and a greater percentage of *KIT* mutations.[45] Targeted therapy with KIT inhibitors is feasible in locally advanced and metastatic cases,[47,48] so evaluation of tumor tissue for *KIT* mutations can be valuable. Subsite differences in mutation patterns can also be seen, such as between vulvar and vaginal melanomas.[49] There is some indication that specific mutations (eg, in *KIT* exons 11 and 13) convey prognostic differences, and whether there are other driver mutations that are unique to mucosal melanoma remains to be determined.

Operative Management

In contrast with cutaneous primary melanomas, the anatomic constraints imposed by the location of most mucosal melanomas limits the extent of excision such that wide margins traditionally achieved on the skin are rarely possible. Reconstructive issues are also far more complex than routinely encountered on the skin. Each site poses its own specific surgical challenges, and discussing them is beyond the scope of this review. A consistent observation, however, has been that more radical operative procedures, such as abdominoperineal resection for anorectal melanoma or radical vulvovaginectomy for vulvar or vaginal melanoma, have never been shown to have an advantage over more conservative procedures.[50–52] This has been most extensively evaluated for anorectal melanoma. A single-institution experience spanning 20 years of cases showed similar results despite a transition away from abdominoperineal resection: Local recurrence was seen in 21% of patients who underwent abdominoperineal resection compared with 26% of those undergoing local excision, with similar 5-year melanoma-specific survival of 34% and 35%, respectively.[50] Similar results were found in a review of 143 patients identified from the national Surveillance, Epidemiology and End Results database. Five-year survival was similar for patients undergoing abdominoperineal resection (16.8%) and local excision (19.3%).[51] Although sentinel lymph node biopsy is feasible in at least some cases of localized mucosal melanoma, available data are simply too limited to draw firm conclusions about its role.[52,53] We currently utilize sentinel node biopsy with single photon emission CT/CT lymphoscintigraphy routinely for anal, perianal, and vulvar melanomas, but are more selective in pursuing sentinel node biopsy for true mucosal melanomas (rectal, vaginal, and nasal/oropharyngeal sites).

Adjuvant Therapy

The limitations of radical surgery for mucosal melanoma have increased the emphasis on adjuvant therapy approaches, especially the use of adjuvant radiation.[54,55] Radiation is used frequently after maximal surgery in most cases of mucosal melanoma and, although randomized data are nonexistent, in-field recurrences seem to be reduced with its use. The value of systemic therapy is even less well studied. A randomized phase II trial in Chinese patients with mucosal melanoma, undoubtedly the largest prospective trial ever conducted in this disease, showed that treatment with either IFN or temozolomide/cisplatin chemotherapy resulted in improved outcomes compared with surgery alone.[56] Surprisingly, given the experience in other types of melanoma, adjuvant chemotherapy in this study was associated with the best relapse-free and overall survival outcomes. This observation, however, requires further validation before adjuvant chemotherapy can be considered a standard for this type of melanoma.

MELANOMA ARISING IN THE EYE

Ocular melanomas include those arising on the conjunctiva, iris, ciliary body, and choroid. Most ocular melanomas arise from uveal melanocytes (the uveal tract includes the iris, ciliary body, and choroid, and is distinct from the pigment cells of the retinal epithelium), although conjunctival melanomas account for only about 5% to 10% of cases.[57] The epidemiology of ocular melanoma is poorly understood, and it remains controversial how much of a role exposure to ultraviolet radiation plays in the development of melanoma at different sites within the eye.[58] Still, there is evidence to point to ultraviolet exposure as etiologic in the eye just as on the skin: Susceptibility factors include light eye color, fair skin, an inability to tan, and chronic sun exposure.[59] Quantifying to role of ultraviolet exposure is complicated by the difficulty in measuring how much ultraviolet radiation different parts of the eye receive, which is far more complex a task than measuring skin exposure. For example, fair-skinned individuals with light eye color may have extensive sun exposure to their skin and a high risk of developing cutaneous melanoma, yet because they routinely wear sunglasses and a hat or cap have very little cumulative sun exposure on and inside their eyes. Another area that has hindered our understanding of ocular melanoma in comparison with cutaneous melanoma is that many ocular primaries are diagnosed noninvasively and treated in place. Thus, the full range of histopathologic prognostic features that can be evaluated on biopsy tissue in cutaneous melanoma are often unavailable for ocular primaries, and early diagnosis of very small melanomas in the eye is quite challenging. New data regarding the genetics of ocular melanoma have potential long-term implications for management and raise issues that so far have not been addressed in cutaneous melanoma.

Site-Specific Differences

It stands to reason that melanomas on or near the surface of the eye (conjunctiva, iris, and ciliary body) would present with different signs and symptoms than those arising deep within the globe. These more superficial tumors are also usually easier to diagnose and biopsy than the deeper lesions. Choroidal melanomas are often asymptomatic and unrecognized until they have grown to a substantial size, when they can be manifest as a persistent blind spot or irregular astigmatism, or be seen on direct ophthalmoscopy during a routine medical or ophthalmic examination. As discussed, genetic differences also exist between melanomas arising within different sites in the eye.

Relevant Biology

For choroidal melanomas, *BRAF* mutations are extremely uncommon. Instead, the MAP kinase pathway seems to be activated through mutations in so-called G-coupled proteins like GNAQ[60] and GNA11.[61] In addition, choroidal melanomas frequently exhibit a loss of the BRCA-associated protein 1 (*BAP1*) gene.[62] Importantly, *BAP1* loss as well as other genetic abnormalities such as monosomy of chromosome 3 have clear prognostic significance in choroidal melanoma.[63,64] This led to the development of a commercially available gene expression profile (GEP) test for choroidal melanoma; using multivariate analysis, GEP class had a stronger independent association with metastasis than any other prognostic factor.[64] Conjunctival melanomas, in contrast to choroidal melanoma, have a mutation pattern much closer to cutaneous melanoma, with frequent *BRAF* mutations.[57] Recently, it has been shown that BRAF mutant conjunctival melanomas can respond to BRAF inhibitor therapy.[65]

Just as has occurred in cutaneous melanoma, expanding our understanding of the genetic basis of sporadic ocular melanomas led to discoveries about inherited melanoma syndromes. Germline mutations in *BAP1* have been found to result in a syndrome including development of choroidal melanoma, cutaneous melanoma, mesothelioma, and other nonmelanocytic malignancies, as well as atypical Spitzoid tumors.[66,67] Importantly, the atypical Spitzoid tumors in these familial cases can be histologically quite bizarre, so recognition of the syndrome is important to avoid overdiagnosis of multiple melanomas in affected patients.

Operative Management

Conjunctival, iris, and ciliary body melanomas are treated by surgery when complete removal is compatible with continued eyesight, but this is rarely possible for choroidal melanomas. Most choroidal melanomas are treated by plaque radiotherapy, with a radioactive plaque implanted surgically for a period of days or weeks to deliver an ablative dose of radiation to the primary while sparing as much of the surrounding retina and optic nerve as possible.[68] Very large ocular melanomas, and those in eyes that have already lost their sight, are managed by enucleation. Most of the eye is not supplied with lymphatics, so regional lymph node metastases are not seen and sentinel lymph node biopsy has no role in the management of choroidal melanoma. An exception is conjunctival melanoma, where nodal metastases do occur and where limited experience has suggested that sentinel node biopsy, although more difficult and complex than for cutaneous primaries, can be performed and can identify micrometastatic disease within the regional lymph nodes.[69]

Adjuvant Therapy and Operative Management of Metastatic Disease

Most adjuvant therapy trials in melanoma have excluded all patients with ocular melanoma, and there are few current data to suggest that adjuvant IFN would be of value for these patients.[70] Nonetheless, the availability of a GEP test that identifies many choroidal melanoma patients as being at high risk of distant metastasis has led more ocular melanoma patients than ever before to seek evaluation for adjuvant therapy. At present, however, the optimal management of choroidal melanoma patients after primary therapy based on GEP class is totally unknown. The preferred approach is enrollment of patients into a clinical trial, with GEP class used as a stratification factor. Unfortunately, few if any such studies are currently available.

Choroidal melanoma has a propensity to metastasize preferentially to the liver, which is often the only site of metastasis in this disease. Unfortunately, the metastatic pattern is usually diffuse and multifocal throughout the liver, so resection of 1 or a few isolated liver metastases from an ocular primary is rarely feasible, even in high-volume centers.[71] Surgical oncologists may yet have a key role to play in the management of liver-predominant metastatic melanoma, using percutaneous hepatic perfusion with intraarterial chemotherapy.[72,73]

SUMMARY

Roughly 1 in 10 cases of melanoma presents as a rare form of the disease with distinct biologic characteristics that impart unique clinical and pathologic features. Awareness of the features that distinguish key subtypes – melanoma of unknown primary, pediatric melanoma, and mucosal and ocular melanoma – informs the pathologic workup and clinical decision making. Surgical decisions should be tailored by knowledge of differences in outcomes and challenges related to patient age and primary tumor location. Choices for adjuvant therapy and treatment of metastatic disease are informed by distinct molecular subclasses in some instances. Despite advances in knowledge about melanoma in general, the relative rarity of these subtypes makes studies of optimum diagnostic modalities and treatment challenging, and future research should focus on prospective and retrospective examination of large cohorts of these patients with long-term follow-up. Until then, surgeons will be called on to evaluate and treat melanoma patients presenting in these unusual fashions using knowledge gained from experience both with the specific situation and generalized from all other melanoma cases as well.

ACKNOWLEDGMENTS

The authors thank K.B. Simons, MD, Professor of Ophthalmology and Pathology, Associate Dean for Graduate Medical Education and Accreditation, Medical College of Wisconsin, Milwaukee, Wisconsin, for helpful feedback and critique of the section on melanomas arising in the eye.

REFERENCES

1. Chang AE, Hynds Karnell L, Menck HR. The National Cancer Data Base report on cutaneous and noncutaneous melanoma. A summary of 84,836 cases from the past decade. Cancer 1998;83:1664–78.
2. Wong JR, Harris JK, Rodriguez-Galindo C, et al. Incidence of childhood and adolescent melanoma in the United States: 1973-2009. Pediatrics 2013;131:846–54.
3. Cormier JN, Xing Y, Feng L, et al. Metastatic melanoma to lymph nodes in patients with unknown primary sites. Cancer 2006;106:2012–20.
4. Lee CC, Faries MB, Wanek L, et al. Improved survival after lymphadenectomy for nodal metastasis from an unknown primary melanoma. J Clin Oncol 2008; 26:535–41.
5. Egberts F, Bergner I, Krüger S, et al. Metastatic melanoma of unknown primary resembles the genotype of cutaneous melanomas. Ann Oncol 2014;25:246–50.
6. Sondak VK, Tuthill R, Moon J, et al. Should unknown primary melanomas be excluded from adjuvant trials? Insights from SWOG S0008. J Clin Oncol 2010; 28:15S (Suppl I):615s.
7. Weide B, Faller C, Elsässer M, et al. Melanoma patients with unknown primary site or nodal recurrence after initial diagnosis have a favourable survival compared to those with synchronous lymph node metastasis and primary tumour. PLoS One 2013;8:e66953.
8. Kirkwood JM, Manola J, Ibrahim J, et al. A pooled analysis of Eastern Cooperative Oncology Group and intergroup trials of adjuvant high-dose interferon for melanoma. Clin Cancer Res 2004;10:1670–7.
9. Eggermont AM, Suciu S, Testori A, et al. Long-term results of the randomized phase III trial EORTC 18991 of adjuvant therapy with pegylated interferon alfa-2b versus observation in resected stage III melanoma. J Clin Oncol 2012; 30:3810–8.
10. Mocellin S, Lens MB, Pasquali S, et al. Interferon alpha for the adjuvant treatment of cutaneous melanoma. Cochrane Database Syst Rev 2013;(6):CD008955.
11. Burmeister BH, Henderson MA, Ainslie J, et al. Adjuvant radiotherapy versus observation alone for patients at risk of lymph-node field relapse after therapeutic lymphadenectomy for melanoma: a randomised trial. Lancet Oncol 2012;13: 589–97.
12. Hauschild A, Grob JJ, Demidov LV, et al. Dabrafenib in BRAF-mutated metastatic melanoma: a multicentre, open-label, phase 3 randomised controlled trial. Lancet 2012;380:358–65.
13. McArthur GA, Chapman PA, Robert C, et al. Safety and efficacy of vemurafenib in BRAF V600E and BRAF V600K mutation-positive melanoma (BRIM-3): extended follow-up of a phase 3, randomised, open-label study. Lancet Oncol 2014;15: 323–32.
14. Flaherty KT, Infante JR, Daud A, et al. Combined BRAF and MEK inhibition in melanoma with BRAF V600 mutations. N Engl J Med 2012;367:1694–703.
15. Hamid O, Robert C, Daud A, et al. Safety and tumor responses with lambrolizumab (anti–PD-1) in melanoma. N Engl J Med 2013;369:134–44.

16. Wolchok JD, Kluger H, Callahan MK, et al. Nivolumab plus ipilimumab in advanced melanoma. N Engl J Med 2013;369:122–33.
17. Swetter SM, Ecker PM, Johnson DL, et al. Primary dermal melanoma. A distinct subtype of melanoma. Arch Dermatol 2004;140:99–103.
18. Balch CM, Gershenwald JE, Soong S-J, et al. Final version of 2009 AJCC melanoma staging and classification. J Clin Oncol 2009;27:6199–206.
19. Cassarino DS, Cabral ES, Kartha RV, et al. Primary dermal melanoma: distinct immunohistochemical findings and clinical outcome compared with nodular and metastatic melanoma. Arch Dermatol 2008;144:49–56.
20. Lyle PL, Amato CM, Fitzpatrick JE, et al. Gastrointestinal melanoma or clear cell sarcoma? Molecular evaluation of 7 cases previously diagnosed as malignant melanoma. Am J Surg Pathol 2008;32:858–66.
21. Lee CC, Faries MB, Wanek L, et al. Improved survival for stage IV melanoma from an unknown primary site. J Clin Oncol 2009;27:3489–95.
22. Council on Environmental Health. Ultraviolet radiation: a hazard to children and adolescents. Pediatrics 2011;127:588–97.
23. Balk SJ, Fisher DE, Geller AC. Teens and indoor tanning: a cancer prevention opportunity for pediatricians. Pediatrics 2013;131:772–85.
24. Gerami P, Busam K, Cochran A, et al. Histomorphologic assessment and inter-observer diagnostic reproducibility of atypical Spitzoid melanocytic neoplasms with long-term follow-up. Am J Surg Pathol 2014;38:934–40.
25. Reed D, Kudchadkar R, Zager JS, et al. Controversies in the evaluation and management of atypical melanocytic proliferations in children, adolescents, and young adults. J Natl Compr Canc Netw 2013;11:679–86.
26. Livestro DP, Kaine EM, Michaelson JS, et al. Melanoma in the young: differences and similarities with adult melanoma. A case-matched controlled analysis. Cancer 2007;110:614–24.
27. Coit DG, Ernstoff MS, Busam KJ. Is pediatric melanoma always malignant? Cancer 2013;119:3910–3.
28. Lange JR, Palis BE, Chang DC, et al. Melanoma in children and teenagers: an analysis of patients from the National Cancer Data Base. J Clin Oncol 2007;25:1363–8.
29. Han D, Zager JS, Han G, et al. The unique clinical characteristics of melanoma diagnosed in children. Ann Surg Oncol 2012;19:3888–95.
30. Averbook BJ, Lee SJ, Delman KA, et al. Pediatric melanoma: analysis of an international registry. Cancer 2013;119:4912–9.
31. Cordero KM, Gupta D, Frieden IJ, et al. Pediatric melanoma: results of a large cohort study and proposal for modified ABCD detection criteria for children. J Am Acad Dermatol 2013;68:913–25.
32. Pearce MS, Salotti JA, Little MP, et al. Radiation exposure from CT scans in childhood and subsequent risk of leukaemia and brain tumors: a retrospective cohort study. Lancet 2012;380:499–505.
33. Berg P, Wennberg AM, Tuominen R, et al. Germline CDKN2A mutations are rare in child and adolescent cutaneous melanoma. Melanoma Res 2004;14:251–5.
34. Daniotti M, Ferrari A, Fregerio S, et al. Cutaneous melanoma in childhood and adolescence shows frequent loss of INK4A and gain of KIT. J Invest Dermatol 2009;129:1759–68.
35. Gerami P, Zembowicz A. Update on fluorescence in situ hybridization in melanoma: state of the art. Arch Pathol Lab Med 2011;135:830–7.
36. Gerami P, Cooper C, Bajaj S, et al. Outcomes of atypical Spitz tumors with chromosomal copy numbers aberrations and conventional melanomas in children. Am J Surg Pathol 2013;37:1387–94.

37. Conway C, Beswick S, Elliott F, et al. Deletion at chromosome arm 9p in relation to BRAF/NRAS mutations and prognostic significance for primary melanoma. Genes Chromosomes Cancer 2010;49:425–38.

38. Gerami P, Scolyer RA, Xu X, et al. Risk assessment for atypical spitzoid melanocytic neoplasms using FISH to identify chromosomal copy number aberrations. Am J Surg Pathol 2013;37:676–84.

39. Ludgate MW, Fullen DR, Lee J, et al. The atypical Spitz tumor of uncertain biologic potential: a series of 67 patients from a single institution. Cancer 2009;115:631–41.

40. Mills OL, Marzban S, Zager JS, et al. Sentinel node biopsy in atypical melanocytic neoplasms in childhood: a single institution experience in 24 patients. J Cutan Pathol 2012;39:331–6.

41. Kirkwood JM, Jukic DM, Averbook BJ, et al. Melanoma in pediatric, adolescent, and young adult patients. Semin Oncol 2009;36:419–31.

42. Cao MM, Schwartz JL, Wechsler DS, et al. High-risk surgically resected pediatric melanoma and adjuvant interferon therapy. Pediatr Blood Cancer 2004;43:1–8.

43. Navid F, Furman WL, Fleming M, et al. The feasibility of adjuvant interferon alpha-2b in children with high-risk melanoma. Cancer 2005;103:780–7.

44. Daud AI, Xu C, Hwu WJ, et al. Pharmacokinetic/pharmacodynamics analysis of adjuvant pegylated interferon α-2b in patients with resected high-risk melanoma. Cancer Chemother Pharmacol 2010;67:657–66.

45. Curtin JA, Busam K, Pinkel D, et al. Somatic activation of KIT in distinct subtypes of melanoma. J Clin Oncol 2006;24:4340–6.

46. Koomen ER, de Vries E, van Kempen LC, et al. Epidemiology of extracutaneous melanoma in the Netherlands. Cancer Epidemiol Biomarkers Prev 2010;19: 1453–9.

47. Bastian BC, Esteve-Puig R. Targeting activated KIT signaling for melanoma therapy. J Clin Oncol 2013;31:3288–90.

48. Minor DR, Kashani-Sabet M, Garrido M, et al. Sunitinib therapy for melanoma patients with KIT mutations. Clin Cancer Res 2012;18:1457–63.

49. Aulmann S, Sinn HP, Penzel R, et al. Comparison of molecular abnormalities in vulvar and vaginal melanomas. Mod Pathol 2014. [Epub ahead of print].

50. Yeh JJ, Shia J, Hwu WJ, et al. The role of abdominoperineal resection as surgical therapy for anorectal melanoma. Ann Surg 2006;244:1012–7.

51. Iddings DM, Fleisig AJ, Chen SL, et al. Practice patterns and outcomes for anorectal melanoma in the USA, reviewing three decades of treatment: is more extensive surgical resection beneficial in all patients? Ann Surg Oncol 2010; 17:40–4.

52. Sugiyama VE, Chan JK, Kapp DS. Management of melanomas of the female genital tract. Curr Opin Oncol 2008;20:565–9.

53. Kobayashi K, Ramirez PT, Kim EE, et al. Sentinel node mapping in vulvovaginal melanoma using SPECT/CT lymphoscintigraphy. Clin Nucl Med 2009;34: 859–61.

54. Christopherson K, Malyapa RS, Werning JW, et al. Radiation therapy for mucosal melanoma of the head and neck. Am J Clin Oncol 2013. [Epub ahead of print].

55. Bishop KD, Olszewski AJ. Epidemiology and survival outcomes of ocular and mucosal melanomas: a population-based analysis. Int J Cancer 2014;134: 2961–71.

56. Lian B, Si L, Cui C, et al. Phase II randomized trial comparing high-dose IFN-α2b with temozolomide plus cisplatin as systemic adjuvant therapy for resected mucosal melanoma. Clin Cancer Res 2013;19:4488–98.

57. Griewank KG, Westekemper H, Murali R, et al. Conjunctival melanomas harbor BRAF and NRAS mutations and copy number changes similar to cutaneous and mucosal melanomas. Clin Cancer Res 2013;19:3143–52.
58. Hu D, McCormick SA. Progress in the studies of etiology, epidemiology and pathogenesis of ocular melanomas. Eye Sci 2011;26:18–22.
59. Shields CL. The hunt for the secrets of uveal melanoma. Clin Experiment Ophthalmol 2008;36:277–80.
60. Van Raamsdonk CD, Bezrookove V, Green G, et al. Frequent somatic mutations of GNAQ in uveal melanoma and blue naevi. Nature 2009;457:599–602.
61. Van Raamsdonk CD, Griewank KG, Crosby MB, et al. Mutations in GNA11 in uveal melanoma. N Engl J Med 2010;363:2191–9.
62. Harbour JW, Onken MD, Roberson ED, et al. Frequent mutation of BAP1 in metastasizing uveal melanomas. Science 2010;330:1410–3.
63. Shields CL, Ganguly A, Bianciotto CG, et al. Prognosis of uveal melanoma in 500 cases using genetic testing of fine-needle aspiration biopsy specimens. Ophthalmology 2011;118:396–401.
64. Onken MD, Worley LA, Char DH, et al. Collaborative Ocular Oncology Group report number 1: prospective validation of a multi-gene prognostic assay in uveal melanoma. Ophthalmology 2012;119:1596–603.
65. Weber JL, Smalley KS, Sondak VK, et al. Conjunctival melanomas harbor BRAF and NRAS mutations—letter. Clin Cancer Res 2013;19:6329–30.
66. Njauw CN, Kim I, Piris A, et al. Germline BAP1 inactivation is preferentially associated with metastatic ocular melanoma and cutaneous-ocular melanoma families. PLoS One 2012;7:e35295.
67. Busam KJ, Wanna M, Wisener T. Multiple epithelioid Spitz nevi or tumors with loss of BAP1 expression. A clue to a hereditary tumor syndrome. JAMA Dermatol 2013;49:335–9.
68. Murray TG, Markoe AM, Gold AS, et al. Long-term followup comparing two treatment dosing strategies of (125)I plaque radiotherapy in the management of small/medium posterior uveal melanoma. J Ophthalmol 2013;2013:517032.
69. Cohen VM, Tsimpida M, Hungerford JL, et al. Prospective study of sentinel lymph node biopsy for conjunctival melanoma. Br J Ophthalmol 2013;97:1525–9.
70. Lane AM, Egan KM, Harmon D, et al. Adjuvant interferon therapy for patients with uveal melanoma at high risk of metastasis. Ophthalmology 2009;116:2206–12.
71. Ryu SW, Saw R, Scolyer RA, et al. Liver resection for metastatic melanoma: equivalent survival for cutaneous and ocular primaries. J Surg Oncol 2013; 108:129–35.
72. Forster MR, Rashid OM, Perez MC, et al. Chemosaturation with percutaneous hepatic perfusion for unresectable metastatic melanoma or sarcoma to the liver: a single institution experience. J Surg Oncol 2014;109:434–9.
73. Agarwala SS, Eggermont AM, O'Day S, et al. Metastatic melanoma to the liver: a contemporary and comprehensive review of surgical, systemic, and regional therapeutic options. Cancer 2014;120:781–9.

Surgical Treatment Options for Stage IV Melanoma

Iris H. Wei, MD, Mark A. Healy, MD, Sandra L. Wong, MD, MS*

KEYWORDS

- Metastasis • Melanoma • Stage IV melanoma • Metastasectomy
- Melanoma surgery

KEY POINTS

- Metastatic melanoma is classified as M1a, M1b, or M1c disease, based on the location of metastasis.
- Melanomas have unique tumor biology and unpredictable patterns of metastasis.
- Prognostic factors for metastatic melanoma include site of metastasis, number of metastatic lesions, and disease-free interval from the time of primary resection.
- In carefully selected patients, there is a survival benefit to metastasectomy.
- Surgical resection of metastatic melanoma may be performed for curative or palliative intent. Candidates for surgical resection generally have favorable prognostic factors.
- Targeted biologic therapies (eg, vemurafenib, dabrafenib, trametinib) and immunomodulatory therapies (eg, antibodies to *CTLA-4* and *PD-1*, adoptive cell transfer) are promising new treatments associated with improved progression-free and overall survival. In the setting of new, effective medical therapies, further study is needed to determine how best to combine nonsurgical and surgical treatments for stage IV melanoma.

INTRODUCTION

Stage IV melanoma is defined by the presence of distant metastasis. Approximately 4% of all melanoma cases are classified as stage IV, and patients have an overall 5-year survival of approximately 5% to 10% and a median survival of 6 to 10 months, depending on the extent and location of metastasis.[1] The overall poor prognosis of metastatic melanoma is partly caused by its unique tumor biology and its tendency to metastasize unpredictably to virtually any organ site. The seventh edition of the

The authors have nothing to disclose.
Department of Surgery, University of Michigan, 1500 East Medical Center Drive, Ann Arbor, MI 48109, USA
* Corresponding author.
E-mail address: wongsl@umich.edu

American Joint Committee on Cancer (AJCC) divides M1 disease into 3 categories, based on the location of metastasis (**Table 1**).[2] There are significant prognostic differences between the groups, with a 3-year survival rate of 30% in patients with M1a disease, compared with 20% in M1b and 15% in M1c disease.[3]

A significant survival benefit has been shown for metastasectomy in highly selected patients with stage IV melanoma undergoing resection, with 5-year survival rates typically ranging from 15% to 30%, depending on the extent of disease and tumor biology.[4-7] Although based primarily on retrospective data, these findings have recently been confirmed in 2 large-scale, prospective studies. In the phase II Southwest Oncology Group (SWOG) study, patients with stage IV melanoma were prospectively followed with serial imaging every 6 months after metastasectomy until disease relapse and death.[8] After complete surgical resection, these patients achieved an overall survival of 21 months. The Malignant Melanoma Active Immunotherapy Trial for stage IV disease (MMAIT-IV) study was a phase III trial randomizing patients with completely resected metastatic melanoma to adjuvant treatment with allogeneic whole-cell vaccine (Canvaxin) plus bacille Calmette-Guerin (BCG) or placebo plus BCG.[9,10] Although there was no difference in outcomes between the two groups, the study population had an overall 5-year survival rate of 42.3%, which is the highest ever achieved in the setting of complete metastasectomy.

Surgical resection in patients with metastatic melanoma has increased in recent years, from an estimated 13% in 2000% to 30% in 2007.[11] Although the data to support incomplete resection, or debulking, in the treatment of melanoma are unclear, a significant number of patients nonetheless benefit from resection for palliation.[12] Decision making for resection is multifactorial. Medical therapies often require multiple treatments to achieve any clinical effect, whereas resection can yield a complete response in a short time frame with little morbidity.[4] In addition, some medical treatments may induce tumor resistance over time, but surgical resection may be repeated in select circumstances with significant clinical benefit.[4,13] Although some degree of micrometastasis and circulating tumor cells likely remain after intended curative resection,[14,15] resection can also limit the progression of melanoma, through several immune-mediated mechanisms. Surgical cytoreduction decreases the amount of tumor-secreted immunosuppressant factors[7] and may also help to promote normal host immune function. By decreasing the tumor burden on the overwhelmed antitumor response system, more antitumor antibodies and lymphocytes are made available to eradicate residual disease.[7,16]

PREOPERATIVE PLANNING

Surgical resection for metastatic melanoma may be performed with curative or palliative intent. During the preoperative evaluation, a thorough history and physical

Table 1		
AJCC M1 classification		
Classification	Site	Serum LDH
M1a	Distant skin, subcutaneous tissue, or lymph node	Normal
M1b	Lung	Normal
M1c	All other visceral metastases	Normal
	Any distant metastasis	Increased

Abbreviation: LDH, lactate dehydrogenase.
Data from Edge S, Byrd DR, Compton CC, et al, editors. AJCC cancer staging manual. 7th edition. New York: Springer; 2010.

examination must be performed; important factors to consider include underlying comorbidities, performance status, and anticipated survival.[2] Appropriate candidates for surgical resection have limited disease burden. Measurement of serum lactate dehydrogenase (LDH) may also help stratify some patients, because increased serum LDH, which characterizes M1c disease, is an important predictor of poor outcome in stage IV melanoma.[17,18] To evaluate additional sites of metastases in patients with stage IV melanoma, computed tomography (CT) of the chest, abdomen, and pelvis should be performed, along with brain magnetic resonance imaging.[19] Symptoms also direct further evaluation. For example, dedicated ultrasonography can be used to assess suspicious lymph node basins,[20] and nuclear medicine bone scans are considered to evaluate patients with complaints of bony pain.[4] 18-Fluorodeoxyglucose (FDG) positron emission tomography (PET)–CT may also be used to identify occult metastases, although small pulmonary lesions, lymph node deposits, and intracranial metastases may be missed (**Fig. 1**).[21–24]

Important factors to consider before surgical resection are the potential for aggressive behavior of metastatic lesions and the likelihood of favorable outcome with

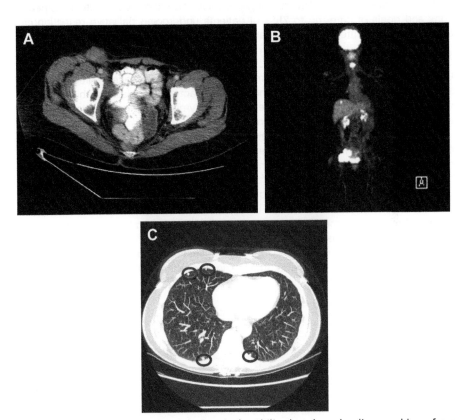

Fig. 1. Metastatic disease to the right inguinal and iliac lymph nodes, liver, and lung from a right thigh melanoma. Four years after wide resection of the primary melanoma, this 66-year-old woman presented with a right groin mass. (A) Pelvic CT showed metastatic disease to her right inguinal and iliac lymph nodes. (B) These lymph nodes were FDG-avid on full-body PET scan, which also identified hypermetabolic lesions in the liver and lung. (C) Subsequent thin-cut chest CT revealed innumerable bilateral pulmonary nodules (*red circles*), which had not been visualized on the PET scan.

resection. Patients with fewer sites of metastatic disease have better outcomes; median survival after resection for a patient with a single metastatic lesion is 29 months, but, if more than 3 sites are involved, survival decreases to 14 months.[13,25,26] It has previously been shown that tumor growth rate, as measured by tumor-volume doubling time, is inversely correlated with patient prognosis and survival.[27,28] The disease-free interval is a commonly used proxy for tumor growth rate and has consistently been shown to be an important predictor of long-term survival. Patients presenting with metastatic disease within the first year of diagnosis have much worse outcomes than those with longer disease-free periods.[13,29,30]

Most patients with metastatic melanoma do not fulfill criteria to be considered appropriate candidates for curative resection. However, resection with palliative intent should be contemplated in those patients with significant bleeding, bowel obstruction, or other tumor-related effects (eg, pain, neurologic symptoms). Palliative resection should especially be considered if the operation is straightforward and offers reasonable success for alleviating symptoms. A detailed conversation about the potential risks and benefits of resection must be had by the patient, family members, and multidisciplinary care team.[21] With careful patient selection and clearly defined expectations and goals of care, up to 75% of patients undergoing palliative resection can be successfully treated, with reasonable associated morbidity.

Surgery for M1a Disease

Up to 40% of patients with stage IV melanoma have M1a disease.[29] Median survival after complete resection is 18 to 40 months.[25,26] Factors associated with better prognosis are skin and soft tissue disease (vs distant lymph node metastasis), fewer and smaller lesions, and longer disease-free interval.[30]

Treatment of distant lymph node metastasis includes complete dissection of the corresponding lymph node basin when possible.[31] For skin and soft tissue metastasis, resection with wide margins is preferred, because disease can infiltrate along tissue planes beyond the palpable mass.[2,4] Skin and subcutaneous metastases can often present as a diffuse process that requires extensive tissue resection (**Fig. 2**). In patients in whom soft tissue metastasis is too bulky or locally advanced to be amenable to local resection, chemotherapy administered via isolated limb perfusion or infusion may be considered if disease is confined to an extremity.[32–34]

Immunotherapy administered by topical application of imiquimod or by intralesional injection of BCG, interferon, interleukin-2, or other investigational agents (eg,

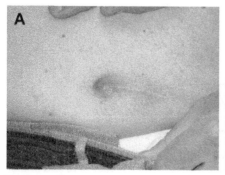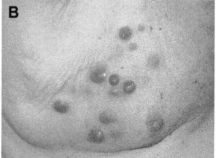

Fig. 2. Locally recurrent cutaneous melanoma with M1a metastases. This patient presented with recurrent disease of the lateral abdominal wall (*A*), as well as distant skin and subcutaneous metastases along the anterior chest (*B*).

Allovectin-7, OncoVEX^{GM-CSF}, PV-10 [known as rose bengal]) has been used in the treatment of cutaneous and subcutaneous melanoma metastases.[35–39] In addition to local tumor ablation, a systemic adjuvant response to local therapy, or bystander effect, has been seen. Direct therapeutic injections into metastatic lesions are thought to be associated with a local reduction in tumor burden, concomitant with immunologic activation. As such, there is potential for combining systemic treatment with intralesional therapies, and clinical trials are emerging to evaluate this.

Patients who achieve partial or complete response to therapy should be reevaluated for definitive surgical resection at all sites.[4] With complete resection of M1a disease, 35-month to 60-month overall survival is reported.[13,40]

Surgery for M1b Disease

The lungs are the most common site of visceral metastases, comprising 15% to 35% of patients with metastatic melanoma.[41,42] Although melanoma tends to follow unpredictable patterns of metastasis, one study reported that among patients with melanoma, there is a 10% annual risk of developing pulmonary metastases at 5 years and a 30% annual risk at 20 years.[41] Some pulmonary metastases do not cause symptoms and may be incidentally found on chest radiograph or CT scan. However, the role of routine radiologic surveillance is controversial, because a recent prospective study showed that surveillance chest radiographs for patients with micrometastatic nodal disease only successfully identified half of patients who developed pulmonary metastases.[43] In patients who received routine chest radiographs, there was no difference in time to detection of metastatic disease or long-term outcomes; there was a significant risk of morbidity from extensive work-ups for false-positive findings.

Multiple studies have shown improved survival after pulmonary metastasectomy, with median survival from 10 to 28 months and 5-year survival rates up to 14% to 35% (from 4%).[5,26,40,44,45] Positive prognostic factors include complete resection, disease-free interval greater than 1 year, fewer than 3 pulmonary nodules, absence of extrathoracic and lymph node metastasis, and response to chemotherapy/immunotherapy.[41,46]

Although multiple and even bilateral pulmonary nodules are not considered technical contraindications to resection,[45] baseline pulmonary status must be carefully evaluated. Surgical principles include adequate resection margins with maximal preservation of normal lung parenchyma.[1] Open or minimally invasive approaches may be considered. Patients rarely develop metastases to the trachea, larynx, or bronchus, and present with cough or hemoptysis. Treatment in these cases includes endoscopic fulguration, external beam radiation, and selective use of pneumonectomy.[47]

Surgery for M1c Disease

Gastrointestinal tract

Gastrointestinal (GI) metastases are rare sites of melanoma, occurring in 2% to 4% of patients with melanoma. However, among metastatic tumors to the GI tract, melanoma is the most common primary tumor, accounting for one-third of all metastases.[21] The most common sites of GI metastases are the small bowel, colon, and stomach.[1] These patients are commonly symptomatic and often present with intractable symptoms of bowel obstruction, GI bleeding, pain, or weight loss.[21] Such patients are often considered for palliative resection even if complete resection is not possible. With appropriate patient selection, palliation may be successfully achieved in 79% to 97% of symptomatic patients.[48–52]

As with other sites of melanoma metastasis, complete resection of GI disease is associated with improved overall survival. Compared with nonsurgical treatment, patients undergoing complete resection of GI metastases have increased median survival from 6 to 48 months.[6] With surgical resection, 5-year survival rates are improved to 38% to 41%,[21,53,54] even in patients with synchronous metastatic sites.[51] Favorable prognostic factors include normal LDH, disease-free interval longer than 2 years, and solitary visceral lesions.[52]

Central nervous system

Melanoma is the third most common source of metastatic lesions to the central nervous system (CNS). More than half of patients with metastatic melanoma develop clinically detectable brain metastases, and 60% of these become symptomatic,[1,55,56] manifesting as headache, seizure, neurologic deficits, or behavioral changes.[21,57] Cerebral metastases account for 20% to 54% of deaths from melanoma, and as many as 75% of patients with metastases have brain involvement at the time of death.[39,57] Presence of brain metastasis portends a poor prognosis, with overall survival of 3 to 7 months.[58,59] Treatment options include surgical resection, whole-brain radiation therapy (WBRT), and stereotactic radiosurgery (SRS).[4] With complete surgical resection, 85% of patients achieve tumor control, and survival can be increased to as much as 22 months.[60–62] Even patients with multiple brain metastases may benefit from surgery if complete resection can be achieved, with outcomes comparable with those patients with single lesions; however, the morbidity of possible neurologic sequelae must be considered before resection.[63] Factors associated with increased survival include a single lesion, younger age, good performance status, lack of neurologic symptoms, and absence of extracranial disease.[2] Because risk of recurrent CNS disease can be as high as 50%, resection is often followed by WBRT.[64]

WBRT can improve neurologic symptoms in two-thirds of patients but confers no survival benefit when used alone.[65] Two randomized controlled trials have shown that patients with single brain metastases from melanoma and other primary cancers have improved survival, lower risk of recurrence, and improved functional quality of life when they receive treatment in an adjuvant setting.[66,67]

SRS is an effective treatment option for patients with melanoma with multiple brain metastases or isolated lesions smaller than 3.5 cm.[60,68] The technique involves delivery of high-dose radiation to targeted regions.[69] SRS has been shown to provide an 83% to 86% tumor control rate and a median survival of 5 to 10 months in experienced centers.[70,71] Although a phase II randomized study comparing WBRT with SRS plus WBRT showed no difference in overall survival, the combination of treatment modalities did improve local tumor control.[72]

Metastasis to the spinal cord is rare but can be extremely morbid.[73] Patient factors must be carefully considered when deciding between the primary treatment options of external beam radiation versus surgical decompression. In a recent randomized controlled trial comparing radiation with surgery in patients with compressive, metastatic spinal lesions from melanoma and other primary tumors, surgically treated patients had improved duration of ambulation, continence, and other outcomes.[74]

Liver

Hepatic metastases most commonly arise from ocular melanomas, which lack adjacent lymphatics and therefore metastasize hematogenously.[75] In contrast, cutaneous melanomas typically spread to the regional lymph nodes, soft tissues, and lungs.[76]

Surgical resection There are no randomized studies investigating the role of resection in treating melanoma metastases to the liver, but retrospective case series suggest a significant survival benefit.[77] Compared with nonsurgical therapy, median overall survival has been reported to increase from between 3 and 12 months to between 14 and

24 months in patients with ocular melanoma[78–80] and from 6 months to 28 months in cutaneous melanoma cases.[81] Multiple studies have consistently shown that survival is most significantly improved by the ability to achieve complete resection.[77–79,82,83]

Regional therapies Regional therapies directed to the liver allow the delivery of intensified treatment, while limiting systemic toxicity. These techniques include hepatic intra-arterial (HIA) chemotherapy, chemoembolization, and isolated or percutaneous hepatic perfusion.[77] In HIA chemotherapy, catheters are introduced into the hepatic artery via the gastroduodenal artery surgically[84,85] or the femoral artery percutaneously,[86–89] and chemotherapy (fotemustine, melphalan, cisplatin) is administered over 3 to 8 treatments. In various retrospective and phase I and II trials, response rates have ranged from 16% to 36%, with a median overall survival of 9 to 21 months.[84–86,88,89] One randomized phase III trial compared HIA with systemic fotemustine in previously untreated, unresectable hepatic metastases from ocular melanoma.[90] Although the response rate was higher in HIA versus systemic chemotherapy (11% vs 2%), there was no difference in overall survival, and the trial was stopped early because of futility.

Hepatic arterial embolization is another technique for delivering directed, high-dose treatment (chemotherapy, immunotherapy, or radiotherapy), followed by an embolic agent to induce selective ischemia.[77] Studies investigating transarterial chemoembolization have reported response rates up to 39% and overall survival of 5 to 8.9 months.[91–95] Important prognostic factors are extent of liver involvement, additional visceral metastases, and baseline LDH.[91–94]

Another regional technique for treating hepatic metastases is hepatic perfusion; access is obtained either surgically or percutaneously. In isolated hepatic perfusion, the vascular supply is surgically isolated and controlled.[96] The most commonly used chemotherapeutic agent is melphalan, an alkalyating agent with optimal pharmacokinetics, including a short exposure time.[97] There have been 3 noncomparative studies investigating metastatic hepatic disease from ocular melanomas, showing tumor response rates of 33% to 62% and overall survival of 10 to 12 months, although disease progression was common and the procedure was associated with considerable morbidity and prolonged hospitalization.[98–100]

Percutaneous hepatic perfusion (PHP) was developed to avoid the morbidity of an open operation, as well as to allow the possibility for repeated treatments.[77] In this technique, the femoral artery is percutaneously accessed and melphalan is administered directly into the hepatic artery. The retrohepatic inferior vena cava is isolated via a double balloon catheter and the blood filtered extracorporeally before being returned to the systemic circulation via an internal jugular vein catheter. A randomized controlled phase III trial of PHP has recently been completed in patients with unresectable hepatic metastases, comparing PHP-delivered melphalan every 4 to 8 weeks with best alternative care. Preliminary results show an improved progression-free survival of 8.1 months in patients receiving PHP, compared with 1.6 months in controls.[101]

Other sites of disease
Splenectomy may be considered as a palliative measure for treatment of pain related to splenic metastases.[21] One study examining splenectomy in a small group of patients with solitary splenic lesions showed improved survival of 20 months, compared with 7 months in those patients treated nonsurgically.[102] Survival benefit has also been shown for resection of adrenal metastases, compared with patients managed nonoperatively.[103] In contrast, pancreatic resection may be performed for palliative benefit,

but there has been no clear evidence that doing so improves long-term survival.[54] In rare cases, intracardiac metastases have been reported, with palliative resection performed to prevent thromboembolic complications.[104]

SURGERY AS ADJUVANT THERAPY

Recent advances in understanding of the molecular and genetic mechanisms that drive tumorigenesis and induce immune tolerance in melanoma have led to the development of several successful immunotherapies and oncogene-targeted therapies. These advances may lead to a reinterpretation of the role of surgical resection in the treatment of metastatic melanoma. Responses to these agents are typically rapid and can be sustained, making them good candidates for neoadjuvant therapy.

Studies using immune-modulating antibodies to target critical regulators of the immune system (CTLA-4, PD-1, PDL1, CD40, CD137, and OX40) have yielded promising results in select patients with metastatic melanoma.[105] Although ipilimumab, an anti–CTLA-4 antibody, produces only a 10% to 15% tumor response rate, long-term survival in responders can be prolonged, with 20% of patients surviving beyond 5 years.[106,107] MK3475, a PD-1 antibody, similarly produced a 38% to 52% response rate, which was independent of prior failure of ipilimumab therapy; there was also improved progression-free survival of greater than 6 months.[108]

Other therapeutic targets are the genes BRAF, NRAS, and CKIT, which play important roles in tumor initiation, progression, and metastasis,[109] and in which driver mutations are present in 60% to 70% of cutaneous melanomas. In patients with these activating mutations (which are tested for to determine eligibility for treatment), targeted therapy using such agents as the US Food and Drug Administration (FDA)–approved BRAF inhibitors vemurafenib and dabrafenib have been shown to improve survival, compared with conventional chemotherapy.[110] However, in the case of BRAF-targeted therapy, clinical resistance can develop approximately 6 to 7 months after initiation of treatment.[111–113] The subsequent discovery of MAPK-dependent mechanisms of resistance have led to the targeting of the downstream MAPK pathway, such as with the FDA-approved MAPK kinase (MEK) inhibitor trametinib, to optimize therapy in patients with BRAF-dependent melanoma.[114–117] Treating multiple targets is now the focus of several studies; most recently, Flaherty and colleagues[118] showed that combined BRAF and MEK inhibition improved both tumor response and progression-free survival compared with monotherapy.

Although no standard chemotherapy treatments have shown improvement in overall survival, several agents are used for palliation. Dacarbazine (DTIC) is the only FDA-approved chemotherapy agent for the treatment of metastatic melanoma, producing a response rate of 10% to 15%, through inhibition of DNA synthesis.[58,119] Temozolomide offers an orally administered, activated formulation of DTIC, producing similar effects with improved CNS penetration.[120] Other chemotherapeutic agents include paclitaxel, cisplatin, carboplatin, and vinblastine, which are used in combination with other biologic agents (eg, interleukin-2, interferon-alfa) and show improved tumor response rates and progression-free survival compared with chemotherapy alone.[121] However, these studies have failed to show significant increases in overall survival.

Adoptive cell transfer (ACT) is a novel technique by which the autologous T lymphocytes of a patient with cancer are isolated and expanded in vitro, then reinfused into the patient after administration of a lymphodepleting chemotherapy, which is used to boost antitumor activity.[122] Compared with biologic and other immunomodulatory therapies, these personalized cancer vaccines can theoretically overcome the immunosuppressive tumor microenvironment. In a study of patients with otherwise medically refractory metastatic melanoma, ACT produced partial or complete tumor regression in 51% of the patients.[123] Although the results are promising, a major obstacle of this treatment is that it is a labor-intensive, personalized therapy requiring laboratory expertise that is unavailable to most clinicians, and therefore most patients.[122]

Neoadjuvant therapy is used in the treatment of several cancers, prolonging survival in bladder, breast, cervical, and esophageal cancers. Surgical outcomes are also improved in breast, laryngeal, and colorectal cancers when neoadjuvant therapy is given; such advantages have occasionally been shown in cases of metastatic disease, in which up-front systemic treatments have allowed curative-intent resection. Medical therapies should be considered in cases of nonresectable metastatic melanoma, with a goal of achieving locoregional control or disease response.[124] In addition, melanoma harbors a unique immunogenicity, in which the normal, cytotoxic T-cell–mediated antitumor response is overwhelmed by tumor-induced immune-evasive mechanisms late in the course of disease. This process suggests that, in the case of melanoma treatment, up-front immunotherapy may favorably alter the disease course. A recent prospective trial studying the use of up-front ipilimumab in patients with stage IIIB/C melanoma showed a significant increase in regulatory and effector T cells, while decreasing myeloid-derived suppressor cells.[125] These immunomodulatory changes correlated with improved progression-free survival, suggesting that ipilimumab may provide an important advantage in altering the tumor microenvironment when used in the neoadjuvant setting.

SUMMARY

Tumor biology and careful patient selection are important in determining the role of surgical resection in patients with stage IV melanoma. In highly selected patients, resection of metastatic disease can provide significant palliation or improved survival. Continued work is needed to determine how best to combine nonsurgical treatments with metastasectomy to further improve patient outcomes.

REFERENCES

1. Leung AM, Hari DM, Morton DL. Surgery for distant melanoma metastasis. Cancer J 2012;18:176–84.
2. Edge SB, Compton CC. The American Joint Committee on Cancer: the 7th edition of the AJCC cancer staging manual and the future of TNM. Ann Surg Oncol 2010;17:1471–4.
3. Balch CM, Soong SJ, Atkins MB, et al. An evidence-based staging system for cutaneous melanoma. CA Cancer J Clin 2004;54:131–49.
4. Martinez SR, Young SE. A rational surgical approach to the treatment of distant melanoma metastases. Cancer Treat Rev 2008;34:614–20.
5. Neuman HB, Patel A, Hanlon C, et al. Stage-IV melanoma and pulmonary metastases: factors predictive of survival. Ann Surg Oncol 2007;14:2847–53.
6. Panagiotou I, Brountzos EN, Bafaloukos D, et al. Malignant melanoma metastatic to the gastrointestinal tract. Melanoma Res 2002;12:169–73.
7. Morton DL, Ollila DW, Hsueh EC, et al. Cytoreductive surgery and adjuvant immunotherapy: a new management paradigm for metastatic melanoma. CA Cancer J Clin 1999;49:101–16, 65.
8. Sosman JA, Moon J, Tuthill RJ, et al. A phase 2 trial of complete resection for stage IV melanoma: results of Southwest Oncology Group Clinical Trial S9430. Cancer 2011;117:4740–6.

9. Rosenthal R, Viehl CT, Guller U, et al. Active specific immunotherapy phase III trials for malignant melanoma: systematic analysis and critical appraisal. J Am Coll Surg 2008;207:95–105.

10. Morton DL, Mozzillo N, Thompson JA, et al. An international, randomized, double-blind, phase 3 study of the specific active immunotherapy agent, Onamelatucel-L (Canvaxin), compared to placebo as post-surgical adjuvant in AJCC stage IV melanoma. Ann Surg Oncol 2006;13(2 Suppl):5s.

11. Huo J, Du XL, Lairson DR, et al. Utilization of surgery, chemotherapy, radiation therapy, and hospice at the end of life for patients diagnosed with metastatic melanoma. Am J Clin Oncol 2013. [Epub ahead of print].

12. Wargo JA, Tanabe K. Surgical management of melanoma. Hematol Oncol Clin North Am 2009;23:565–81, x.

13. Ollila DW, Hsueh EC, Stern SL, et al. Metastasectomy for recurrent stage IV melanoma. J Surg Oncol 1999;71:209–13.

14. Koyanagi K, Kuo C, Nakagawa T, et al. Multimarker quantitative real-time PCR detection of circulating melanoma cells in peripheral blood: relation to disease stage in melanoma patients. Clin Chem 2005;51:981–8.

15. Koyanagi K, Mori T, O'Day SJ, et al. Association of circulating tumor cells with serum tumor-related methylated DNA in peripheral blood of melanoma patients. Cancer Res 2006;66:6111–7.

16. Hsueh EC, Gupta RK, Yee R, et al. Does endogenous immune response determine the outcome of surgical therapy for metastatic melanoma? Ann Surg Oncol 2000;7:232–8.

17. Balch CM, Buzaid AC, Soong SJ, et al. New TNM melanoma staging system: linking biology and natural history to clinical outcomes. Semin Surg Oncol 2003;21:43–52.

18. Franzke A, Probst-Kepper M, Buer J, et al. Elevated pretreatment serum levels of soluble vascular cell adhesion molecule 1 and lactate dehydrogenase as predictors of survival in cutaneous metastatic malignant melanoma. Br J Cancer 1998;78:40–5.

19. National Comprehensive Cancer Network. Melanoma (version 3.2014). NCCN clinical practice guidelines in oncology. Available at: www.nccn.org. Accessed July 30, 2014.

20. Garbe C, Paul A, Kohler-Spath H, et al. Prospective evaluation of a follow-up schedule in cutaneous melanoma patients: recommendations for an effective follow-up strategy. J Clin Oncol 2003;21:520–9.

21. Wong SL, Coit DG. Role of surgery in patients with stage IV melanoma. Curr Opin Oncol 2004;16:155–60.

22. Cobben DC, Koopal S, Tiebosch AT, et al. New diagnostic techniques in staging in the surgical treatment of cutaneous malignant melanoma. Eur J Surg Oncol 2002;28:692–700.

23. Mijnhout GS, Hoekstra OS, van Lingen A, et al. How morphometric analysis of metastatic load predicts the (un)usefulness of PET scanning: the case of lymph node staging in melanoma. J Clin Pathol 2003;56:283–6.

24. Spieth K, Risse J, Kaufmann R, et al. Challenging cases and diagnostic dilemmas: case 3. Positron emission tomography scan mimicking lymph node metastases in a high-risk melanoma patient. J Clin Oncol 2002;20:3349–51.

25. Essner R. Surgical treatment of malignant melanoma. Surg Clin North Am 2003; 83:109–56.

26. Essner R, Lee JH, Wanek LA, et al. Contemporary surgical treatment of advanced-stage melanoma. Arch Surg 2004;139:961–6 [discussion: 966–7].

27. Joseph WL, Morton DL, Adkins PC. Prognostic significance of tumor doubling time in evaluating operability in pulmonary metastatic disease. J Thorac Cardiovasc Surg 1971;61:23–32.

28. Ollila DW, Stern SL, Morton DL. Tumor doubling time: a selection factor for pulmonary resection of metastatic melanoma. J Surg Oncol 1998;69:206–11.

29. Ollila DW. Complete metastasectomy in patients with stage IV metastatic melanoma. Lancet Oncol 2006;7:919–24.

30. Wong JH, Skinner KA, Kim KA, et al. The role of surgery in the treatment of nonregionally recurrent melanoma. Surgery 1993;113:389–94.

31. Mack LA, McKinnon JG. Controversies in the management of metastatic melanoma to regional lymphatic basins. J Surg Oncol 2004;86:189–99.

32. Knorr C, Meyer T, Janssen T, et al. Hyperthermic isolated limb perfusion (HILP) in malignant melanoma. Experience with 101 patients. Eur J Surg Oncol 2006; 32:224–7.

33. Noorda EM, Vrouenraets BC, Nieweg OE, et al. Prognostic factors for survival after isolated limb perfusion for malignant melanoma. Eur J Surg Oncol 2003; 29:916–21.

34. Sanki A, Kam PC, Thompson JF. Long-term results of hyperthermic, isolated limb perfusion for melanoma: a reflection of tumor biology. Ann Surg 2007; 245:591–6.

35. Green DS, Bodman-Smith MD, Dalgleish AG, et al. Phase I/II study of topical imiquimod and intralesional interleukin-2 in the treatment of accessible metastases in malignant melanoma. Br J Dermatol 2007;156:337–45.

36. Nathanson L. Regression of intradermal malignant melanoma after intralesional injection of *Mycobacterium bovis* strain BCG. Cancer Chemother Rep 1972;56: 659–65.

37. Tan JK, Ho VC. Pooled analysis of the efficacy of bacille Calmette-Guerin (BCG) immunotherapy in malignant melanoma. J Dermatol Surg Oncol 1993;19:985–90.

38. Wolf IH, Smolle J, Binder B, et al. Topical imiquimod in the treatment of metastatic melanoma to skin. Arch Dermatol 2003;139:273–6.

39. Ito F, Chang AE. Cancer immunotherapy. Current status and future directions. Surg Oncol Clin N Am 2013;22:765–83.

40. Batus M, Waheed S, Ruby C, et al. Optimal management of metastatic melanoma: current strategies and future directions. Am J Clin Dermatol 2013;14: 179–94.

41. Harpole DH Jr, Johnson CM, Wolfe WG, et al. Analysis of 945 cases of pulmonary metastatic melanoma. J Thorac Cardiovasc Surg 1992;103:743–8 [discussion: 748–50].

42. Pogrebniak HW, Stovroff M, Roth JA, et al. Resection of pulmonary metastases from malignant melanoma: results of a 16-year experience. Ann Thorac Surg 1988;46:20–3.

43. Morton RL, Craig JC, Thompson JF. The role of surveillance chest X-rays in the follow-up of high-risk melanoma patients. Ann Surg Oncol 2009;16:571–7.

44. Schuhan C, Muley T, Dienemann H, et al. Survival after pulmonary metastasectomy in patients with malignant melanoma. Thorac Cardiovasc Surg 2011;59: 158–62.

45. Caudle AS, Ross MI. Metastasectomy for stage IV melanoma: for whom and how much? Surg Oncol Clin N Am 2011;20:133–44.

46. Tafra L, Dale PS, Wanek LA, et al. Resection and adjuvant immunotherapy for melanoma metastatic to the lung and thorax. J Thorac Cardiovasc Surg 1995; 110:119–28 [discussion: 129].

47. Koyi H, Branden E. Intratracheal metastasis from malignant melanoma. J Eur Acad Dermatol Venereol 2000;14:407–8.
48. Agrawal S, Yao TJ, Coit DG. Surgery for melanoma metastatic to the gastrointestinal tract. Ann Surg Oncol 1999;6:336–44.
49. Berger AC, Buell JF, Venzon D, et al. Management of symptomatic malignant melanoma of the gastrointestinal tract. Ann Surg Oncol 1999;6:155–60.
50. Khadra MH, Thompson JF, Milton GW, et al. The justification for surgical treatment of metastatic melanoma of the gastrointestinal tract. Surg Gynecol Obstet 1990;171:413–6.
51. Ollila DW, Essner R, Wanek LA, et al. Surgical resection for melanoma metastatic to the gastrointestinal tract. Arch Surg 1996;131:975–9, 979–80.
52. Ricaniadis N, Konstadoulakis MM, Walsh D, et al. Gastrointestinal metastases from malignant melanoma. Surg Oncol 1995;4:105–10.
53. Chua TC, Saxena A, Morris DL. Surgical metastasectomy in AJCC stage IV M1c melanoma patients with gastrointestinal and liver metastases. Ann Acad Med Singapore 2010;39:634–9.
54. Sanki A, Scolyer RA, Thompson JF. Surgery for melanoma metastases of the gastrointestinal tract: indications and results. Eur J Surg Oncol 2009;35:313–9.
55. Grob JJ, Regis J, Laurans R, et al. Radiosurgery without whole brain radiotherapy in melanoma brain metastases. Club de Cancerologie Cutanee. Eur J Cancer 1998;34:1187–92.
56. Mingione V, Oliveira M, Prasad D, et al. Gamma surgery for melanoma metastases in the brain. J Neurosurg 2002;96:544–51.
57. Sampson JH, Carter JH Jr, Friedman AH, et al. Demographics, prognosis, and therapy in 702 patients with brain metastases from malignant melanoma. J Neurosurg 1998;88:11–20.
58. Fox MC, Lao CD, Schwartz JL, et al. Management options for metastatic melanoma in the era of novel therapies: a primer for the practicing dermatologist: part II: Management of stage IV disease. J Am Acad Dermatol 2013;68: 13.e1–13.
59. Fife KM, Colman MH, Stevens GN, et al. Determinants of outcome in melanoma patients with cerebral metastases. J Clin Oncol 2004;22:1293–300.
60. McWilliams RR, Brown PD, Buckner JC, et al. Treatment of brain metastases from melanoma. Mayo Clin Proc 2003;78:1529–36.
61. Skibber JM, Soong SJ, Austin L, et al. Cranial irradiation after surgical excision of brain metastases in melanoma patients. Ann Surg Oncol 1996;3: 118–23.
62. Tarhini AA, Agarwala SS. Management of brain metastases in patients with melanoma. Curr Opin Oncol 2004;16:161–6.
63. Ewend MG, Carey LA, Brem H. Treatment of melanoma metastases in the brain. Semin Surg Oncol 1996;12:429–35.
64. Oredsson S, Ingvar C, Stromblad LG, et al. Palliative surgery for brain metastases of malignant melanoma. Eur J Surg Oncol 1990;16:451–6.
65. Broadbent AM, Hruby G, Tin MM, et al. Survival following whole brain radiation treatment for cerebral metastases: an audit of 474 patients. Radiother Oncol 2004;71:259–65.
66. Patchell RA, Tibbs PA, Walsh JW, et al. A randomized trial of surgery in the treatment of single metastases to the brain. N Engl J Med 1990;322:494–500.
67. Vecht CJ, Haaxma-Reiche H, Noordijk EM, et al. Treatment of single brain metastasis: radiotherapy alone or combined with neurosurgery? Ann Neurol 1993;33:583–90.

68. Chen JC, Petrovich Z, O'Day S, et al. Stereotactic radiosurgery in the treatment of metastatic disease to the brain. Neurosurgery 2000;47:268–79 [discussion: 279–81].
69. Cattell E, Kelly C, Middleton MR. Brain metastases in melanoma: a European perspective. Semin Oncol 2002;29:513–7.
70. Gaudy-Marqueste C, Regis JM, Muracciole X, et al. Gamma-Knife radiosurgery in the management of melanoma patients with brain metastases: a series of 106 patients without whole-brain radiotherapy. Int J Radiat Oncol Biol Phys 2006;65: 809–16.
71. Mathieu D, Kondziolka D, Cooper PB, et al. Gamma knife radiosurgery in the management of malignant melanoma brain metastases. Neurosurgery 2007; 60:471–81 [discussion: 481–2].
72. Andrews DW, Scott CB, Sperduto PW, et al. Whole brain radiation therapy with or without stereotactic radiosurgery boost for patients with one to three brain metastases: phase III results of the RTOG 9508 randomised trial. Lancet 2004;363:1665–72.
73. Gokaslan ZL, Aladag MA, Ellerhorst JA. Melanoma metastatic to the spine: a review of 133 cases. Melanoma Res 2000;10:78–80.
74. Patchell RA, Tibbs PA, Regine WF, et al. Direct decompressive surgical resection in the treatment of spinal cord compression caused by metastatic cancer: a randomised trial. Lancet 2005;366:643–8.
75. Yonekawa Y, Kim IK. Epidemiology and management of uveal melanoma. Hematol Oncol Clin North Am 2012;26:1169–84.
76. Leiter U, Meier F, Schittek B, et al. The natural course of cutaneous melanoma. J Surg Oncol 2004;86:172–8.
77. Agarwala SS, Eggermont AM, O'Day S, et al. Metastatic melanoma to the liver: a contemporary and comprehensive review of surgical, systemic, and regional therapeutic options. Cancer 2014;120:781–9.
78. Frenkel S, Nir I, Hendler K, et al. Long-term survival of uveal melanoma patients after surgery for liver metastases. Br J Ophthalmol 2009;93:1042–6.
79. Mariani P, Piperno-Neumann S, Servois V, et al. Surgical management of liver metastases from uveal melanoma: 16 years' experience at the Institut Curie. Eur J Surg Oncol 2009;35:1192–7.
80. Marshall E, Romaniuk C, Ghaneh P, et al. MRI in the detection of hepatic metastases from high-risk uveal melanoma: a prospective study in 188 patients. Br J Ophthalmol 2013;97:159–63.
81. Rose DM, Essner R, Hughes TM, et al. Surgical resection for metastatic melanoma to the liver: the John Wayne Cancer Institute and Sydney Melanoma Unit experience. Arch Surg 2001;136:950–5.
82. Rivoire M, Kodjikian L, Baldo S, et al. Treatment of liver metastases from uveal melanoma. Ann Surg Oncol 2005;12:422–8.
83. Ryu SW, Saw R, Scolyer RA, et al. Liver resection for metastatic melanoma: equivalent survival for cutaneous and ocular primaries. J Surg Oncol 2013;108:129–35.
84. Peters S, Voelter V, Zografos L, et al. Intra-arterial hepatic fotemustine for the treatment of liver metastases from uveal melanoma: experience in 101 patients. Ann Oncol 2006;17:578–83.
85. Siegel R, Hauschild A, Kettelhack C, et al. Hepatic arterial fotemustine chemotherapy in patients with liver metastases from cutaneous melanoma is as effective as in ocular melanoma. Eur J Surg Oncol 2007;33:627–32.
86. Agarwala SS, Panikkar R, Kirkwood JM. Phase I/II randomized trial of intrahepatic arterial infusion chemotherapy with cisplatin and chemoembolization

with cisplatin and polyvinyl sponge in patients with ocular melanoma metastatic to the liver. Melanoma Res 2004;14:217–22.

87. Becker JC, Terheyden P, Kampgen E, et al. Treatment of disseminated ocular melanoma with sequential fotemustine, interferon alpha, and interleukin 2. Br J Cancer 2002;87:840–5.

88. Farolfi A, Ridolfi L, Guidoboni M, et al. Liver metastases from melanoma: hepatic intra-arterial chemotherapy. A retrospective study. J Chemother 2011;23:300–5.

89. Heusner TA, Antoch G, Wittkowski-Sterczewski A, et al. Transarterial hepatic chemoperfusion of uveal melanoma metastases: survival and response to treatment. Rofo 2011;183:1151–60.

90. Leyvraz S, Piperno-Neumann S, Suciu S, et al. Hepatic intra-arterial versus intravenous fotemustine in patients with liver metastases from uveal melanoma (EORTC 18021): a multicentric randomized trial. Ann Oncol 2014;25:742–6.

91. Ahrar J, Gupta S, Ensor J, et al. Response, survival, and prognostic factors after hepatic arterial chemoembolization in patients with liver metastases from cutaneous melanoma. Cancer Invest 2011;29:49–55.

92. Gupta S, Bedikian AY, Ahrar J, et al. Hepatic artery chemoembolization in patients with ocular melanoma metastatic to the liver: response, survival, and prognostic factors. Am J Clin Oncol 2010;33:474–80.

93. Patel K, Sullivan K, Berd D, et al. Chemoembolization of the hepatic artery with BCNU for metastatic uveal melanoma: results of a phase II study. Melanoma Res 2005;15:297–304.

94. Schuster R, Lindner M, Wacker F, et al. Transarterial chemoembolization of liver metastases from uveal melanoma after failure of systemic therapy: toxicity and outcome. Melanoma Res 2010;20:191–6.

95. Sharma KV, Gould JE, Harbour JW, et al. Hepatic arterial chemoembolization for management of metastatic melanoma. AJR Am J Roentgenol 2008;190:99–104.

96. Alexander HR Jr, Butler CC. Development of isolated hepatic perfusion via the operative and percutaneous techniques for patients with isolated and unresectable liver metastases. Cancer J 2010;16:132–41.

97. Vahrmeijer AL, van de Velde CJ, Hartgrink HH, et al. Treatment of melanoma metastases confined to the liver and future perspectives. Dig Surg 2008;25:467–72.

98. Alexander HR, Libutti SK, Bartlett DL, et al. A phase I-II study of isolated hepatic perfusion using melphalan with or without tumor necrosis factor for patients with ocular melanoma metastatic to liver. Clin Cancer Res 2000;6:3062–70.

99. Alexander HR Jr, Libutti SK, Pingpank JF, et al. Hyperthermic isolated hepatic perfusion using melphalan for patients with ocular melanoma metastatic to liver. Clin Cancer Res 2003;9:6343–9.

100. van Iersel LB, Hoekman EJ, Gelderblom H, et al. Isolated hepatic perfusion with 200 mg melphalan for advanced noncolorectal liver metastases. Ann Surg Oncol 2008;15:1891–8.

101. Pingpank JF, Hughes MS, Alexander HR, et al. Percutaneous hepatic perfusion (PHP) vs. best alternative care for patients with melanoma liver metastases: efficacy update of the phase 3 trial (NCT00324727). Eur J Cancer 2011; 47(Suppl1):S653 [abstract: 9304].

102. de Wilt JH, McCarthy WH, Thompson JF. Surgical treatment of splenic metastases in patients with melanoma. J Am Coll Surg 2003;197:38–43.

103. Mittendorf EA, Lim SJ, Schacherer CW, et al. Melanoma adrenal metastasis: natural history and surgical management. Am J Surg 2008;195:363–8 [discussion: 368–9].

104. Messner G, Harting MT, Russo P, et al. Surgical management of metastatic melanoma to the ventricle. Tex Heart Inst J 2003;30:218–20.

105. Ribas A, Hersey P, Middleton MR, et al. New challenges in endpoints for drug development in advanced melanoma. Clin Cancer Res 2012;18:336–41.
106. Hodi FS, O'Day SJ, McDermott DF, et al. Improved survival with ipilimumab in patients with metastatic melanoma. N Engl J Med 2010;363:711–23.
107. Robert C, Thomas L, Bondarenko I, et al. Ipilimumab plus dacarbazine for previously untreated metastatic melanoma. N Engl J Med 2011;364:2517–26.
108. Hamid O, Robert C, Daud A, et al. Safety and tumor responses with lambrolizumab (anti-PD-1) in melanoma. N Engl J Med 2013;369:134–44.
109. Davies H, Bignell GR, Cox C, et al. Mutations of the BRAF gene in human cancer. Nature 2002;417:949–54.
110. Chapman PB, Hauschild A, Robert C, et al. Improved survival with vemurafenib in melanoma with BRAF V600E mutation. N Engl J Med 2011;364:2507–16.
111. Flaherty KT, Puzanov I, Kim KB, et al. Inhibition of mutated, activated BRAF in metastatic melanoma. N Engl J Med 2010;363:809–19.
112. Sosman JA, Kim KB, Schuchter L, et al. Survival in BRAF V600-mutant advanced melanoma treated with vemurafenib. N Engl J Med 2012;366:707–14.
113. Hauschild A, Grob JJ, Demidov LV, et al. Dabrafenib in BRAF-mutated metastatic melanoma: a multicentre, open-label, phase 3 randomised controlled trial. Lancet 2012;380:358–65.
114. Nazarian R, Shi H, Wang Q, et al. Melanomas acquire resistance to B-RAF(V600E) inhibition by RTK or N-RAS upregulation. Nature 2010;468:973–7.
115. Villanueva J, Vultur A, Lee JT, et al. Acquired resistance to BRAF inhibitors mediated by a RAF kinase switch in melanoma can be overcome by cotargeting MEK and IGF-1R/PI3K. Cancer Cell 2010;18:683–95.
116. Shi H, Moriceau G, Kong X, et al. Melanoma whole-exome sequencing identifies V600EB-RAF amplification-mediated acquired B-RAF inhibitor resistance. Nat Commun 2012;3:724.
117. Poulikakos PI, Persaud Y, Janakiraman M, et al. RAF inhibitor resistance is mediated by dimerization of aberrantly spliced BRAF(V600E). Nature 2011;480:387–90.
118. Flaherty KT, Infante JR, Daud A, et al. Combined BRAF and MEK inhibition in melanoma with BRAF V600 mutations. N Engl J Med 2012;367:1694–703.
119. Middleton MR, Grob JJ, Aaronson N, et al. Randomized phase III study of temozolomide versus dacarbazine in the treatment of patients with advanced metastatic malignant melanoma. J Clin Oncol 2000;18:158–66.
120. Quirt I, Verma S, Petrella T, et al. Temozolomide for the treatment of metastatic melanoma: a systematic review. Oncologist 2007;12:1114–23.
121. Eton O, Legha SS, Bedikian AY, et al. Sequential biochemotherapy versus chemotherapy for metastatic melanoma: results from a phase III randomized trial. J Clin Oncol 2002;20:2045–52.
122. Rosenberg SA, Restifo NP, Yang JC, et al. Adoptive cell transfer: a clinical path to effective cancer immunotherapy. Nat Rev Cancer 2008;8:299–308.
123. Dudley ME, Wunderlich JR, Yang JC, et al. Adoptive cell transfer therapy following non-myeloablative but lymphodepleting chemotherapy for the treatment of patients with refractory metastatic melanoma. J Clin Oncol 2005;23:2346–57.
124. Davar D, Tarhini AA, Kirkwood JM. Adjuvant immunotherapy of melanoma and development of new approaches using the neoadjuvant approach. Clin Dermatol 2013;31:237–50.
125. Tarhini AA, Edington H, Butterfield LH, et al. Immune monitoring of the circulation and the tumor microenvironment in patients with regionally advanced melanoma receiving neoadjuvant ipilimumab. PLoS One 2014;9:e87705.

Head and Neck Melanoma

Jerry Cheriyan, MD, MRCS[a], Jessica Wernberg, MD[b,*],
Andrew Urquhart, MD[c]

KEYWORDS

- Head and neck melanoma (HNM) • Parotidectomy • Sentinel lymph node
- Treatment of primary lesion • Treatment of draining lymph node

KEY POINTS

- Wide local excision is the mainstay in the treatment of the primary lesion with consideration given to specific anatomic constraints in head and neck melanoma (HNM).
- Sentinel lymph node biopsy (SLNB) is considered in all lesions with ulceration, mitoses greater than or equal to $1/mm^2$, stage1B or higher, and in all high-risk nonmetastatic melanoma.
- Lymphatic drainage patterns in the head and neck can be atypical and may involve the parotid gland.
- Higher rate of locoregional recurrence has been reported in SLN-negative patients in HNM compared with cutaneous melanoma elsewhere.
- Location of primary, SLNB status, node-positive disease, and the drainage pattern determines the extent of neck dissection and parotidectomy.
- Reconstructive strategy must be considered in multidisciplinary teams with reconstructive surgeons for large head and neck defects.

INTRODUCTION
Epidemiology

It is estimated that melanoma of the head and neck comprises 6% to 25% of all cutaneous melanomas.[1–3] Head and neck melanoma (HNM) is uncommon in patients under 30 years of age and is usually seen in adults older than 70 years.[4] Men are at higher risk of developing HNM than women,[5–7] and the incidence of melanoma of the face and neck is two times greater in men than in women, although the differences

Funding Support: None.
Conflict of Interest: The authors have nothing to disclose.
[a] Department of General Surgery, Marshfield Clinic, 1000 North Oak Avenue, Marshfield, WI 54449, USA; [b] Department of General Surgery/Surgical Oncology, Marshfield Clinic, 1000 North Oak Avenue, Marshfield, WI 54449, USA; [c] Department of Otolaryngology/Head and Neck Surgery, Marshfield Clinic, 1000 North Oak Avenue, Marshfield, WI 54449, USA
* Corresponding author.
E-mail address: wernberg.jessica@marshfieldclinic.org

are smaller in younger age groups.[8] Sixty to 90% of HNMs occur on the face,[3,9] with the scalp, neck, and ears less commonly involved (**Fig. 1**).[10–14] The higher incidence of HNM in relation to total body surface area may be explained by the fact that the head and neck area is more affected by increased exposure to ultraviolet radiation and the higher density of melanocytes in the head and neck.[3,15]

Risk factors for HNM include the following:

- Continuous (occupational) sun exposure
- Higher levels of occupational sun exposure, whereas extremity melanoma was associated with a higher total sun exposure[16,17]
- Lighter skin[17,18]
- Increased number of sunburns
- Nevus count, although a positive association between nevus counts to HNM is weaker than that between nevus counts and trunk or extremity melanoma[17]

CLINICAL PRESENTATION
History

As with cutaneous melanoma at any site on the body, early detection and diagnosis of HNM are vital for effective and timely therapeutic intervention. Approximately half of the time, melanoma is self-discovered, with 26% discovered by medical providers and the rest by family members or others.[19] The most common presenting symptom is color change or growth of a preexisting lesion.[20] Other presenting symptoms include itching, bleeding, ulceration, and pain, or paresthesias that would be a manifestation of late symptoms, occurring in thick melanomas.[20] Patients should be asked about risk factors including sun exposure, history of sunburns, and especially family history, because up to 10% of melanoma cases report a first-degree or second-degree relative with melanoma.[21]

Physical Examination

A meticulous and complete skin examination along with examination of typical and atypical lymphatic drainage basins should be performed, noting the number, type, and characteristics of moles or nevi. The American Cancer Society recommended ABCDEs (asymmetry, border, color, diameter, evolving) provide a simple guideline

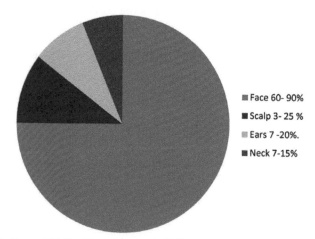

Fig. 1. Distribution of HNMs. (*Data from* Refs.[10–14])

to detect early warning signs of melanoma. Gachon and colleagues[22] suggested the use of the "ugly duckling" warning sign, which focuses on the identification of pigmented or clinically amelanotic lesions that look different from the rest, to assist with the detection of lesions that do not fit the classic ABCDE criteria. Although all of these factors have been found to be predictors of a malignant lesion, an irregular border is the strongest predictor.[23] In the head and neck, particular attention must be devoted to examining the scalp, including the hair-bearing areas, ears, nose, and eyelids in addition to the face. The hair-bearing scalp areas are best examined after taking off all hair bands and clips and then parting the dry loose hair in a systematic fashion using a comb. A complete examination of the ear includes the pinna, the external auditory canal with and without an otoscope, as well as behind the pinna. Both eyelids should be examined when open and closed. Examination of the lymph nodes should include both ipsilateral and contralateral submental, submandibular, jugular, anterior central, and posterior, as well as the supraclavicular and axillary basins.

CLASSIFICATION AND STAGING
Morphology

The morphologic types seen in HNM are similar to cutaneous melanoma. Superficial spreading melanoma is the most common subtype, accounting for 50% to 80% of cases, and appears flat because of the horizontal radial pattern of growth, which is followed by a subsequent vertical growth phase characterized by the presence of a dominant nest in the papillary dermis. Nodular melanoma, accounting for 20% to 30% of cases, is thick on palpation because of early vertical growth of the cancer cells. Lentigo maligna melanoma is commonly seen in later years within preexisting large freckles or Hutchinson freckles (lentigo maligna). Desmoplastic neurotropic melanoma is a variant that often lacks pigment and clinically has characteristics similar to hypertrophic scar, dermatofibroma, or fibrosarcoma with a propensity toward neural invasion. Although it is a rare form of melanoma, accounting for only around 1% of all cases, about half arise in the head and neck.[24]

Histology

The Clark Level and Breslow Thickness are the 2 histologic systems used for classification. Clark grading involves a qualitative system to determine the depth of the primary melanoma based on the level of invasion of the dermis, whereas the Breslow thickness system is based on the quantitative measurement of thickness in millimeters from the stratum granulosum to the deepest point of invasion.[24] The Breslow thickness provides a powerful tool for prognostic staging of melanoma; consequently, emphasis on the Clark system has decreased.

Clinical Staging

Based on current evidence, the American Joint Committee on Cancer has revised the staging for cutaneous melanoma.[25] The latest revision includes ulceration in the scheme and replaces the Clark Level with mitotic rate in thin melanoma, highlighting their association with prognosis. Serum lactate dehydrogenase is included in M classification in addition to defining micrometastases and macrometastases.

INVESTIGATIONS
Biopsy

Excisional biopsy is the preferred technique for small, accessible lesions with a 1-mm to 2-mm margin because it is diagnostic, potentially therapeutic, and prognostic.

Incisional or punch biopsy may be used for sampling larger lesions. Deep shave biopsies are frequently used when lesions are suggestive of both epidermoid carcinoma and melanoma.[24] Needle biopsies are useful for assessing suspicious lymph nodes or metastasis. Careful planning of biopsy orientation is critical in HNM to avoid compromise if subsequent wide local excision and reconstruction becomes indicated.

Imaging Recommendations

The role and extent of imaging for patients with HNM is controversial.[26] Although sentinel lymph node biopsy (SLNB) is not 100% accurate, it is the most reliable means for regional staging and has better sensitivity and specificity than computed tomography (CT), magnetic resonance imaging (MRI), positron emission tomography (PET), elective lymph node dissection (ELND), and clinical examination.[27] There are no recommended routine baseline or surveillance laboratory tests (lactate dehydrogenase, liver function test, chest radiography, CT, MRI, PET, bone scans, or gastrointestinal series) in patients with no signs or symptoms of metastasis. Fluorodeoxyglucose-PET has been shown to be effective for detecting metastatic melanoma, with sensitivity and specificity reported as high as 74% to 100% and 67% to 100%, respectively.[28,29] PET is not recommended in early-stage node-negative HNM, but may be considered if symptoms warrant further imaging or to follow disease burden in stage IV disease.[30]

TREATMENT AND PATHOLOGIC STAGING

The oncologic management is best delivered by a multidisciplinary team, including surgeons, reconstructive surgeons, and medical and radiation oncologists.

Treatment of Primary Lesion

Wide local excision

Wide local excision (WLE) of the index lesion is the primary treatment of cutaneous melanoma. Malignant cells may extend microns to several millimeters beyond clinically visible margins, thus necessitating a wider and frequently deeper excision to ensure as complete a removal as possible. The recommendations for surgical margins for WLE for the head and neck are similar to other cutaneous melanomas, but this is not always possible because of the functional and cosmetic disability that may arise.[31] Historically, a 5-cm margin excision was done until the 1970s, when Breslow and Macht[32] reported successful treatment in thin melanoma patients with narrower margin excision. A prospective randomized control study by the World Health Organization[33] on melanoma concluded that there was no significance in recurrence rates between 1-cm or 3-cm margin resection in cutaneous melanomas 2 mm or less. Surgical margin recommendations from the American Academy of Dermatology (AAD)[34] published in 2011 are based on both evidence from prospective randomized control studies and consensus opinion when no prospective data were available (**Table 1**).

The basis for these recommendations is as follows:

- Wide excision for melanoma is associated with reduced recurrence.
- For thin melanomas, currently there is no high-quality evidence to support excision of more than a 1-cm margin in improving survival or local recurrence rates.
- For primary melanomas of any thickness, there is no evidence to suggest that margin excision of more than 2 cm provides any additional benefit in terms of survival or local recurrence rates.

Table 1
American ADA surgical margin recommendations for primary cutaneous melanoma

Breslow Thickness	Clinically Measured Surgical Margin[a]
In situ	0.5–1.0 cm
≤1 mm	1 cm
1.01–2.0 mm	1–2 cm
>2 mm	2 cm

[a] Wider margins might be necessary for lentigo maligna subtype.
Adapted from Bichakjian CK, Halpern AC, Johnson TM, et al. Guidelines of care for the management of primary cutaneous melanoma. American Academy of Dermatology. J Am Acad Dermatol 2011;65:1032–47.

The AAD also recommends that the depth of excision be carried out to the level of muscle fascia, if possible, or at least to deep adipose tissue depending on location.[34] A wider excision may be considered for lentigo maligna melanoma, given the potential for extensive subclinical extension, particularly in the head and neck.

It is important to note that although the recommendations for surgical margin resection serve as guidelines, margins should be individualized. Adherence to these recommendations might be particularly challenging in HNM because of cosmetic and functional concerns associated with wide excision. Careful consideration of the risk of recurrence, defect size, and location should guide the extent of resection.

Sentinel Node Biopsy and Lymphatic Drainage Patterns

SLNB was introduced by Morton and colleagues[35] and modified by Robinson and colleagues[36] to include preoperative lymphoscintigraphy. SLNB is used to identify the immediate draining lymph node from the primary tumor by injecting radioisotope and or blue dye with or without preoperative lymphoscintigraphy.[37–39] The principle of SLNB is based on the rationale of the primary tumor having defined lymphatic drainage into specific nodal basins with the goal of identifying metastasis to regional lymph nodes. No evidence of metastasis in the sentinel lymph node (SLN) is highly indicative that the remaining nodes will not have metastatic spread.[35] SLNB is the most sensitive and specific staging test for identification of micrometastatic melanoma in regional lymph nodes.[40] As with melanoma of the trunk and extremities, SLNB status is the most important prognostic factor in HNM patients.[31,41,42] SLNB is particularly useful in midline HNM, as lymphatic drainage in the head and neck is often aberrant and can result in identification of the sentinel node in more than one nodal basin or in an atypical, bilateral, or contralateral nodal basin.

Some authors have noted a wide range in the false negative rates (3.4%–10.4%) for HNM SNLB as well as a decreased HNM SLN positive rate (10%–15%) compared with cutaneous melanoma elsewhere (16%–23%).[43,44] Others have reported SLN positive rates in HNM that are not significantly different from other cutaneous melanomas, although the small patient numbers in these studies limit their interpretation. A worse survival in HNM with positive SLN compared with other anatomic locations has also been suggested.[43]

Indications for SLNB

Indications for consideration of SLNB for HNM are similar to those for other cutaneous melanomas and include all patients with lesions that have a Breslow thickness greater than 1.0 mm and a clinically negative nodal basin and all patients with ulceration or an increased mitotic rate (**Fig. 2**). SLNB may be considered for melanoma patients with less than 1.0-mm thickness with adverse features, including positive deep margins, lymphovascular invasion, young patients, or Clark Level IV or greater.[42] Although some prefer not to perform SLNB after WLE due to disruption of natural lymphatic pathways, it may be acceptable even after WLE, if extensive reconstruction and lymphatic dissection have not been performed. One must also be prepared for drainage into atypical, contralateral, and deep cervical lymph node basins.

SLNB technique
Patients are given intradermal injections of a radioactive colloid, usually Technectium-99 sulfur colloid (0.5 mCi), around the primary lesion, after which a lymphoscintigraphy may be performed. If injection of the radiotracer into the subcutaneous tissue results in failure to detect the sentinel node, a repeat injection should be performed. Under anesthesia, intradermal isoflurane blue or methylene blue dye can be injected in addition to the radioactive colloid to map the lymph node. WLE of the melanoma may be performed first to reduce radioactivity from the primary injection, which may interfere with the ability to detect tracer uptake in the SLN; this is especially true in HNM, as the SLN may be in close proximity to the primary lesion. An intraoperative handheld gamma probe is used to localize the SNL and lymphatic channels.[26] Cervical SLNB is performed using a 1-cm to 3-cm incision over the area of maximal radioactivity, while a periauricular incision is usually used for the parotid region. Identification and removal of the sentinel node are performed for all hot lymph nodes until the gamma counts in the basin are equal or less than 10% of the hottest lymph node removed.[40]

Histologic evaluation
Once the SLN is identified and excised, it is recommended that histologic evaluation be done using permanent paraffin section with hematoxylin and eosin staining and immunohistochemistry (IHC), as frozen sections have a high false negative rate ranging from 5% to 10%.[45] Higher sensitivity of the IHC markers S-100 and Melan-A make it the recommended stain compared with HMB-45, which is less sensitive. Permanent section allows for accurately discussing the prognosis and treatment of positive lymphatic nodes with the patient in an office setting before proceeding with definitive treatment.

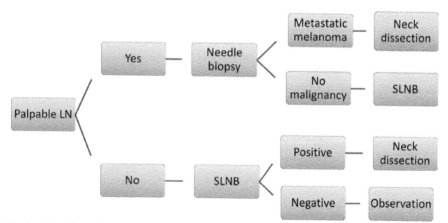

Fig. 2. Algorithm for treatment of lymph node basin in HNMs. LN, lymph node; SLNB, sentinel lymph node biopsy.

ELND

ELND, with the aim of clearing all potential lymph nodes with metastatic melanoma, can have significant morbidity from lymphedema and injury to the major vascular and nervous structures. The survival benefit from ELND in HNM has not been proven, and with findings from the Multicenter Selective Lymphadenectomy trials-I,[37] SLNB has become a more favored approach. A systematic review by Tanis and colleagues[46] concluded that there was no conclusive evidence on the advantage of either elective neck dissection or SLNB in patients with clinically node-negative HNM of intermediate thickness. In a study of 46 patients with metastatic malignant melanoma, the authors concluded that involvement of more than 4 cervical or parotid nodes resulted in significant increase in distant metastases, but did not note an impact of location or metastases or method of neck dissection on survival.[47] Bodem and colleagues[48] suggested that in patients with proven lymph node metastases, complete neck dissection might be of benefit because the number of infiltrated nodes is often higher than expected. The role of neck dissection in HNM is not yet fully established. The number and levels should be determined based on tumor location and SLNB status. Prospective studies are necessary to provide convincing, reliable, and validated guidelines for cervical lymph node dissection in HNM.

Parotid Management

Lymphatic drainage from the face, cheeks, lips, ears, and anterior scalp can include the parotid in addition to the neck. With a primary lesion in this location, the parotid could be a potential source of metastasis, with around 25% to 30% of HNM draining into the parotid lymph node basin.[49,50] Although there is no consensus, the options when lymphoscintigraphy shows drainage to the parotid include parotid-sparing SLNB and superficial parotidectomy followed by cervical lymph node dissection in the event of confirmed metastasis to the SLN. The multiplicity, widespread distribution, and high frequency of parotid nodes have prompted some surgeons to advocate superficial parotidectomy over mapping.[51] Suton and colleagues[52] suggested that parotidectomy be considered for all HNM, except for posterior primaries and lower neck melanomas. Some authors also recommend parotidectomy for anterior melanoma.[53,54] Because of the risk of neurovascular injury to the facial nerve and vessels, others have suggested a targeted, parotid-sparing approach for SLN in the parotid region. The targeted, parotid-sparing approach for SLN is technically more demanding and may place the facial nerve at a higher risk of injury.[55] There are also concerns that fibrosis and inflammation after SLNB might result in an increased risk of facial nerve injury if reoperation of the parotid is necessary. Some studies have reported the low morbidity and accuracy of sentinel lymphadenectomy in the parotid gland.[56,57] Proponents of the parotid lymph node biopsy highlight it as a less invasive operation compared with a superficial parotidectomy, with no increase in recurrence. Although there is a theoretic increased risk of injury to the facial nerve while doing a parotidectomy as a secondary procedure after the SLNB, some groups have noted no increase in facial nerve or bleeding complications.[55] It would be prudent to prepare for a selective lymph node biopsy in the parotid region by an experienced surgeon, while also being prepared to perform a superficial parotidectomy if the SLN is not identified. A parotid lesion can also be investigated with a needle biopsy.

Neck Dissection

Technical aspects

In general, forehead and anterior scalp melanomas spread to the parotid, periparotid, and upper jugular lymph nodes, whereas those in the posterior scalp and occiput spread to the postauricular, suboccipital, and posterior triangle lymph nodes. Melanoma of the face and neck usually metastasize to the facial, submental, submandibular, and deep cervical nodes. The American Head and Neck Society (AHNS) classified the lymph nodes of the neck into 5 levels on each side, a central submental triangle, and a single central compartment (**Fig. 3**). The cheek and eyelid regions have 2 lymphatic drainage patterns, one to the parotid nodes and the other to level IB. The lymph drainage patterns in the lip region are to level IA or IB.[58] Lymphatic drainage of the ear has no predictable pattern, but it most commonly drains to cervical level II and the preauricular and postauricular basins.[59]

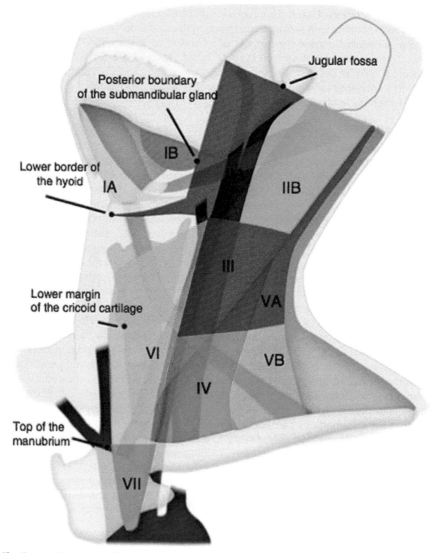

Fig. 3. Level wise classification of neck nodes (Supported by the American Head and Neck Society). (*From* Harisinghani NG. Atlas of lymph node anatomy. New York: Springer; 2013. p. 2; with permission.)

Current guidelines for management of primary cutaneous melanoma do not specify recommendations for HNM.[34] It is justifiable to perform regional lymphadenectomy alone in cases of primaries of the posterior scalp and posterior neck with no involvement of the submandibular and submental triangles.[52]

The AHNS and the American Academy of Otolaryngology-Head and Neck Surgery classified neck dissections into the following:

1. Radical neck dissection (RND)—removal of all ipsilateral cervical lymph node groups from levels I through V, together with spinal accessory nerve, internal jugular vein, and sternocleidomastoid muscle.
2. Modified radical neck dissection (MRND)—removal of all lymph node groups routinely removed in RND, but with preservation of one or more nonlymphatic structures (spinal accessory nerve, internal jugular vein, and sternocleidomastoid muscle).
3. Selective neck dissection (SND)—cervical lymphadenectomy with preservation of one or more lymph node groups and all nonlymphatic structures routinely removed in RND.
4. Extended neck dissection—removal of one or more additional lymph node groups or nonlymphatic structures, or both, not encompassed by RND.

Indications

Neck dissections may be performed in the following clinical scenarios: clinically positive lymph nodes; positive SLNB in the neck; positive SLN in the parotid region; extensive invasive lymph node disease; and clinically negative lymph node disease.

Clinically positive lymph nodes—therapeutic neck dissection Therapeutic lymph node dissection refers to the lymph node removal for clinically evident or palpable lymph nodes. The extent of neck dissection would depend on the number and location of the nodes as well as the primary lesion.

Positive SLNB in the neck—therapeutic neck dissection Completion lymph node dissection is the lymphadenectomy done after a positive SLNB. The extent of neck dissection depends on the level of the SLN and the location of the primary lesion. Gyorki and colleagues[60] reported that positive nonsentinel lymph nodes were mostly identified within or adjacent to the nodal level containing the SLN.

Positive parotid SLN—therapeutic neck dissection and parotidectomy A parotidectomy is indicated with positive parotid SLN as well if clinically apparent disease is present in the parotid. A primary lesion involving the parietal or frontal scalp, face, cheeks, nose, or ear could potentially have drainage to the parotid in addition to the neck; therefore, a parotidectomy should be performed in conjunction with the neck dissection when the SLN is positive.

Extensive invasive lymph node disease—therapeutic neck dissection including nonlymphatic structures RND should only be performed with extensive involvement of the spinal accessory nerve, internal jugular vein, or sternocleidomastoid muscle. There are some data supporting MRND as having comparable efficacy to RND and advantageous efficacy over selective ND[49,61]; however, Shah and colleagues[62] recommend complete RND for therapeutic conditions and limited neck dissection for elective procedures.

No known lymph node disease—elective neck dissection ELND for clinically negative lymph node disease is no longer commonly performed since the advent of SLNB and involves lymph node dissection on patients without palpable lymph nodes or imaging studies suggesting lymph node disease. Proponents of ELND support this option, highlighting the challenges of SLN in the head and neck, especially the parotid region, due to possible atypical as well as multiple drainage patterns, SLN very close to the primary lesion, and the increased incidence of nodal recurrence in SLN negative patients.

ADJUVANT THERAPY
Radiotherapy

There is increased risk of recurrence in neck lymph nodes compared with other lymph node basins, with 24% and 14% recurrence rates in the neck and parotid, respectively.[14] Furthermore, patients who have had recurrence are considered to be at increased risk of further recurrence.[61,63]

Current indications for adjuvant radiotherapy of primary site include[64] HNM, especially mucosal melanomas, desmoplastic neurotropic melanoma, thick melanoma (>4 mm, especially if ulcerated or associated with satellite lesion), and inability to achieve negative resection margin. Lesions close to the eye or central and spinous nervous system can be excluded from radiotherapy.[31] Although adjuvant radiotherapy has been shown to decrease the rate of local recurrence,[65] even for patients with small tumors,[66,67] there are conflicting reports on the effect of radiotherapy on survival.[68,69]

Chemotherapy

Interferon-α-2b (IFN-α-2b) has shown some benefit in patients at high risk of developing distant metastasis,[70] but it has a limited benefit in patients with disseminated melanoma.[71] In patients with nodal metastases, meta-analyses have shown a significant effect of IFN-α-2b on relapse-free survival and small improvements in survival.[72,73]

RECONSTRUCTION

WLE of melanomas of the head and neck can be especially challenging. The need for adequate margin excision is to be carefully balanced with both functional and cosmetic considerations, given the proximity of primary tumor to vital structures like eyes, nose, ears, and lips as well as to nerves and vessels. Also, due consideration should be given to the ease of follow-up examinations for recurrences, as areas at risk may no longer be anatomically oriented after reconstruction.

Reconstruction Timing

Reconstruction can be performed immediately after WLE or may be delayed to ensure negative margins. Because of concerns about recurrence and need for surveillance, delayed reconstruction after WLE has been advised.[74,75] Delayed skin grafting offers advantages of improved recipient bed vascularity, additional tissue bulk, reduced healing time, less contraction, and elimination of adjacent scarring to the defect.[76] Bogle and colleagues[77] found that immediate flap closure when primary closure is not possible can achieve acceptable functional and esthetic results, without compromising detection of recurrence. Immediate reconstruction may be considered in carefully selected patients. Sullivan and colleagues[78,79] suggested that immediate reconstruction is safe for most HNM and did not find any difference in the incidence of positive margins between immediate and delayed reconstruction in 117 patients reviewed. Delayed reconstruction should be undertaken in patients with T4 HNM that is associated with an increased risk of positive margins after WLE, as well as in patients with perineural or bony invasion, or if postoperative radiotherapy is part of the management strategy.

Techniques

Reconstruction options include primary closure, skin graft, local skin flaps, regional muscle or fasciocutaneous flaps, free tissue flaps, tissue expansion, and a combination of one or more of these techniques (**Table 2**).[80–82]

Primary closure, although not always possible, may be performed if the defect is small and incisions are made along relaxing skin tension lines. Types of skin graft used can be full-thickness skin graft (FTSG) and split-thickness skin graft (STSG).

Table 2 Location-specific reconstruction options	
Scalp	
<3 cm	Primary closure
Larger defects	Flaps (transpositional, rotational, rhomboid, V-Y advancement), free tissue transfer, composite reconstruction, skin graft, secondary reconstruction
Forehead	
<2–3 cm	Primary closure
Defects up to 30% involvement	Flaps (transpositional, rotational, rhomboid, V-Y advancement)
Larger defects	Rotational flap, tissue expanders, free tissue transfer
Eyelids	
<One-fourth eyelid	Primary closure
Larger defects	Flaps, skin graft, composite tarsal reconstruction
Lower eyelid	Mustarde-rotation flap
Cheek	
<2 cm	Primary closure
2–4 cm	Rotation or advancement flaps
Large defects	Cervicofacial flaps, fasciocutaneous flaps (radial forearm, lateral arm, parascapular), tissue expander
Lips	
<One-quarter upper lip <One-third lower lip	Primary closure
Lower lip	Webster flap, Karapandzic flap
Upper lip	Abbe flap, Webster perialar advancement technique, Eastlander flap, rhomboid flap
Nose	
Small defect	Full thickness grafts (preauricular, retroauricular, or neck skin), banner, bilobed, dorsal nasal flaps
1.5–2.0 cm or involving nasal subunit	Pedicle flap from the forehead
Amputation of the nose	Prosthesis
Ears	
Small defect	Primary closure
Medium-large defects	FTSG, chondrocutaneous advancement flaps, multistage procedure
Total amputation	Prosthesis

FTSG involves grafting of the epidermis and entire thickness of dermis and is advantageous in that graft characteristics and size are maintained to a greater extent than STSG. This is due to greater collagen content, dermal vasculature, and epithelial appendages preserved in FTSG than STSG.[83] FTSG is especially useful for the face, but has limited applicability to relatively small vascularized wounds and has a higher incidence of graft failure than STSG. Sites of harvest include preauricular and postauricular, clavicular, groin, and buttock regions.[80] STSG involves grafting of epidermis and part of the dermis. Depending on the thickness, STSG can be classified as thin (0.005–0.012 in), intermediate (0.012–0.018 in), or thick (0.018–0.030 in).[84] The thickness of the dermal layer usually depends on the harvest site, age, and gender. STSG can be obtained from any site, but is most commonly harvested from the upper anterior, lateral thigh, or buttock.[84,85] Buttock grafts may cause significant pain and require more harvest site care than other sites. STSG offers the benefit of requiring less than optimal conditions for survival and can be used for large wounds, muscle flaps, mucosal defects, and to line cavities.[84] However, these grafts often do not maintain graft characteristics like color, texture, and hair growth, and they may result in significant contraction, making them less ideal for reconstructions on the face.[84] Furthermore, survivability of STSG after radiation therapy is low. Although graft meshing allows larger surface area coverage and increased take, sheet grafts are preferred for better cosmesis.[80,84]

Local or regional flaps are grafts that have their own blood supply. These flaps may be composite flaps and include cartilage, muscle, bone, and fascia in addition to skin. Local flaps like bilobed, rotational, and rhomboid flaps are primarily used for small defects, whereas regional flaps such as paramedian forehead and nasolabial are used in larger defects.[74] Rhomboid flaps have become increasingly popular for reconstruction of defects in the head and neck region.[24] These flaps are full-thickness grafts that depend on the subdermal vascular plexus for blood supply, rather than axial blood supply.[86] Generally, the pedicle length-to-width in the head and neck ratio is 2 to 4:1 because of the rich vascular network. These flaps are not recommended when there is a possibility of distortion of structures like the eyelid margin or lip due to the resulting tension vectors in rhomboid flaps.[86]

Free tissue transfer is rarely used in HNM reconstruction, but when used, due consideration should be given to caliber of vascular pedicle and recipient site vascular supply. Anterolateral thigh flaps and radial forearm flaps may be used, as these are thin and pliable and facilitate contouring over facial bones.[87–89]

Tissue expansion involves implanting an inflatable silicone tissue expander below tissue that is adjacent to the defect with timed serial expansion of the expander to stimulate new skin. When adequate skin cover has been obtained, the tissue expander is removed, and secondary reconstruction is performed. In complex cases, the use of scaffolds has shown some promise.[90]

Location Specific Reconstructive Options

Scalp

Primary closure can be used for most defects of size less than 3 cm, and skin grafting may be used for larger defects, depending on site characteristics and graftability. A transposition flap, a rotational flap, or a rhomboid transpositional flap may also be options.[80] For reconstruction of large defects in the anterior scalp, superficial temporal fascia pedicled V-Y advancement may be considered. V-Y advancement is advantageous because the flap is very mobile and retains the original hair orientation.[91,92] A temporoparietal-occipital flap can be used to reconstruct anterior hairline defects due to the high length-to-width ratio of the flap (**Fig. 4**).[80] For large defects, skin grafts may be

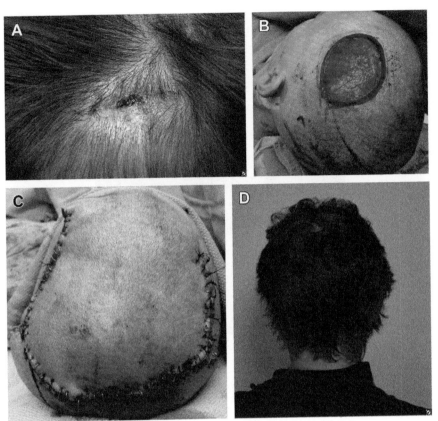

Fig. 4. (*A*) Scalp melanoma. WLE (*B*) and reconstruction (*C*) with rotational scalp flap. (*D*) Postreconstruction.

considered if contour or esthetic considerations are of low priority, because the good pericranial vasculature allows for a favorable take of the graft (**Fig. 5**).[93]

Free-tissue transfers are indicated for very large defects on the scalp vertex or when reconstruction involves bone resection.[74,94] Because of the high possibility of local advancement of melanoma extending to the cranium, resection of the outer cortex or local craniectomy may be necessary. Composite reconstruction using bone grafts or substitutes and flaps are feasible options. A muscle-only flap resurfaced with a split skin graft might be more advantageous than a composite myocutaneous flap because scalp contour is better maintained.[91,95,96] In cases of planned secondary reconstruction, tissue expanders are especially helpful to expand scalp tissue and mobilize tissue for flap advancement, transposition, or rotation.

Forehead
For primary closure of small defects of 2 cm to 3 cm, a vertical elliptical incision is preferred when possible, because it allows for alignment of forehead wrinkles and avoids asymmetry of the eyebrows.[80,91] Skin grafts should be preferably avoided for cosmetic considerations.[91] However, when necessary, clavicular skin-graft should be considered, because it provides a large surface area of skin and has similar characteristics to the skin of the forehead.[93] Rhomboid and advancement flaps can be useful for small defects of the forehead. Rotational flaps are usually used for large

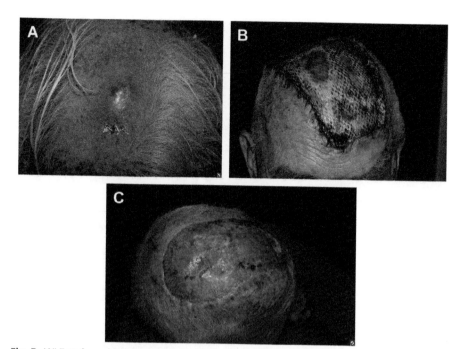

Fig. 5. WLE scalp melanoma (*A*) reconstructed with 160 cm² STSG (*B*). (*C*) Postreconstruction.

defects, with single rotational flaps for lateral defects and bilateral for defects above or near the glabella (**Fig. 6**). A 2-stage reconstruction strategy using tissue expanders may be considered in defects involving 25% to 30% of the forehead. Defects of more than one-third or 50 cm² of the forehead surface area may be best reconstructed using a free-tissue transfer from groin, radial forearm, or scapula.[80,93,95]

Eyelids

Primary closure is possible if the defect is less than one-fourth the lid length with tissue approximation of skin and tarsus.[74] Larger defects require skin grafts or flaps. The lower eyelid can serve as a donor for upper eyelid construction but not vice versa.[97] Multistage lid switch repair is best for large upper eyelid defects.[98] A technique of whole lower lid transfer with the closing of donor site with cheek rotation flap has also been described.[99] Lower eyelid defects can be reconstructed using the Mustarde-rotation flap where tissue is mobilized from the zygoma and temple region. Skin graft of the lower eyelid is not preferred because of the potential complication of ectropion formation.[80] Composite tarsal reconstruction can be performed using the upper lateral cartilage and nasal mucosa, hard palate, or contralateral eyelid.[80] In rare circumstances of local spread of tumor to the globe, orbital exenteration and craniofacial resection may be required.

Cheek

Small defects less than 2 cm in width can usually be closed by primary closure. Rotation or advancement flaps such as the rhomboid, Mustarde, or Esser flap can be used for reconstructing defects between 2 cm and 4 cm (**Fig. 7**). Retraction, scarring, and abnormal contouring may occur with the challenge of orienting the donor site scar along skin tension lines.[80] Cervicofacial flaps are used for larger defect size reconstructions, with free-tissue transfer being a good option for very large defects usually

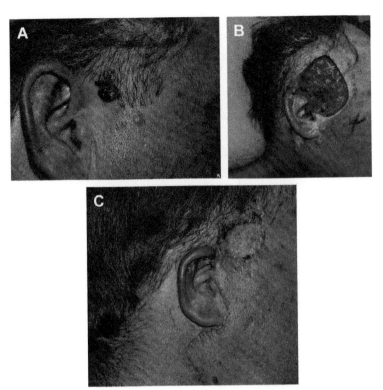

Fig. 6. (*A*) Preauricular melanoma (*B*) WLE involving face, temporal scalp, and upper pole of external ear. (*C*) Reconstruction with antia sliding helical advancement flap, cervical flap, and FTSG.

greater than 10 cm or involving deeper tissues. Fasciocutaneous flaps are excellent for large defects, as they are relatively thin and do not atrophy.[80] Other flaps include radial forearm, lateral arm, and parascapular flap.[80] In cases with facial nerve involvement by the tumor and subsequent resection, a nerve graft may be required; the sural nerve and the contralateral greater auricular nerve are the most common donor nerves. Implantation of tissue expander is a feasible option when secondary reconstruction is planned. It is important to remember that reconstruction should not compromise parotidectomy or neck dissection that may be required in the case of metastatic disease.[91]

Lips

Reconstruction of the lip is technically challenging and requires expertise.[80] With defects involving less than one-quarter of the upper lip or one-third of the lower lip, primary closure may be attempted.[80] It is vital to perform a layered closure of the orbicularis oris, white roll, wet and dry vermillion, and skin. Other lower lip reconstruction techniques include the Webster flap and the Karapandzic flap. The Webster flap involves unilateral or bilateral advancement of full-thickness lip and cheek remnants to close the defect. The Karapandzic flap involves lateral advancement rotation of the cheek and nasolabial skin, with incisions made along the nasolabial and mentolabial creases, making it esthetically more pleasing. The Karapandzic flap, having a neurovascular pedicle, preserves motor and sensory components.[80,91] For upper lip lateral defects, advancement flaps from the adjacent cheek are possible. Abbe flap reconstruction is a two-stage procedure that involves composite tissue from the lower

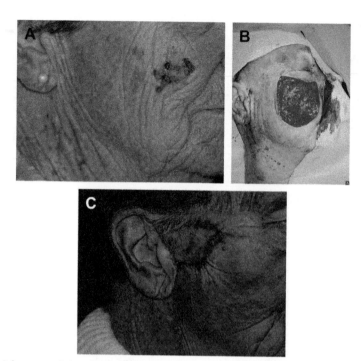

Fig. 7. Melanoma of the cheek (*A*) WLE (*B*) and reconstruction with cervical rotation flap and FTSG (*C*).

lip used to reconstruct the central upper lip. In the first stage, the flap is created along the lateral margin, preserving its pedicle vascular supply and rotating the pedicle onto the upper lip defect. In the second stage, after a few weeks, the flap is divided. Other techniques include the Webster perialar advancement technique, Eastlander flap, and rhomboid flap.[80,91] Microsurgical free-flap transfer can also be attempted for both the upper and the lower lip.

Nose

The role of primary closure in the nose is limited to very small defects. Usually melanoma resections involve only the skin and subcutaneous tissue without extension to framework or mucosal lining.[93] Most melanoma reconstructions require either a local flap or a skin graft. Full-thickness grafts are usually preferred from preauricular, retroauricular, or neck skin.[80] Local flaps are more beneficial, in that they provide better matching color and texture.[80] The Banner, bilobed, and dorsal nasal flaps are commonly used.[100] Defects of 1.5 cm to 2.0 cm or involving more than one nasal subunit are usually resurfaced using a pedicle flap from the forehead (**Fig. 8**).[101–103] The donor site scar should be considered when this technique is used. Under the rare circumstance of local invasion of tumor, a composite reconstruction is required. Prosthesis may be used for total or near total amputation of the nose.[104–106]

Ears

Defects of the ear may be only skin, skin and cartilage (bilaminar), or entire thickness.[80] In cases of small defects limited to just skin, primary closure is possible. Skin grafting might be required if vascularity and cartilage rim is adequate for helical support. Most melanoma lesions arise in the helical rim where it is difficult to perform FTSG.[107] Simple

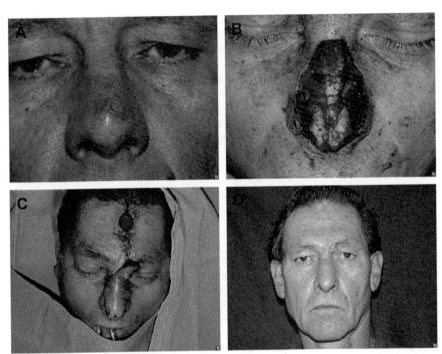

Fig. 8. Nose melanoma (*A*), WLE (*B*) reconstructed with midline forehead flap (*C*). Postreconstruction (*D*).

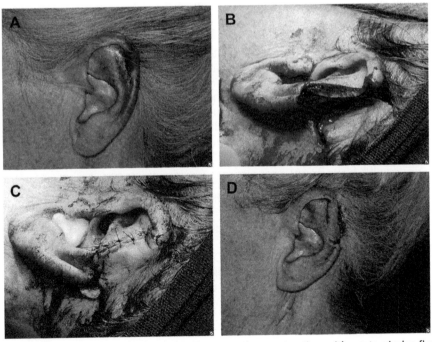

Fig. 9. Melanoma of the external ear (*A*) WLE and reconstruction with postauricular flap and STSG (*B, C*). Postreconstruction (*D*).

wedge excisions with cartilage using Burow's triangles can be used in small defects of the middle or posterior helix.[91,108] Techniques of chondrocutaneous advancement flaps have also been described.[109,110] Wedge excision of melanomas of the middle-third might result in significant asymmetry between ears. Alternatively, a multistage procedure involving burying a cartilage graft under the mastoid skin and advancing it into the auricular defect should be considered (**Fig. 9**).[42] Wedge excision and direct closure are usually sufficient for caudal-third ear lesions. As with nasal reconstructions, a total or near total ear amputation can be reconstructed using a prosthesis, including osseointegrated mastoid clip prosthesis.[111]

Mohs Surgery

There is some indication that Mohs surgery is useful for resection in difficult areas and large-diameter superficial lesions like lentigo maligna.[112,113] However, further investigation is necessary before considering Mohs surgery as standard procedure.[31]

SUMMARY

The management of HNM, although similar to cutaneous melanoma elsewhere, can range from being straightforward to quite formidable. The oncologic resection margins of the primary lesion in HNM must be balanced against the cosmetic and functional outcomes. Lymphatic drainage in the head and neck can be in close proximity to the primary lesion or vital structures and is often atypical, making SLNB technically challenging. Treatment of the draining lymph node region depends on the clinical nodal and SLNB status in addition to the location of the primary lesion. These factors direct the extent of neck dissection and the indications for a parotidectomy. With large defects following resection, the whole gamut of reconstructive options must be explored and individualized to patients' needs.

REFERENCES

1. Myers JN. Value of neck dissection in the treatment of patients with intermediate-thickness cutaneous malignant melanoma of the head and neck. Arch Otolaryngol Head Neck Surg 1999;125:110–5.
2. Lachiewicz AM, Berwick M, Wiggins CL, et al. Epidemiologic support for melanoma heterogeneity using the surveillance, epidemiology, and end results program. J Invest Dermatol 2008;128:1340–2.
3. Hoersch B, Leiter U, Garbe C. Is head and neck melanoma a distinct entity? A clinical registry-based comparative study in 5702 patients with melanoma. Br J Dermatol 2006;155:771–7.
4. Ciocan D, Barbe C, Aubin F, et al. Distinctive features of melanoma and its management in elderly patients: a population-based study in france. JAMA Dermatol 2013;149:1150–7.
5. Shashanka R, Smitha BR. Head and neck melanoma. ISRN Surg 2012;2012:948302.
6. Franklin JD, Reynolds VH, Bowers DG Jr, et al. Cutaneous melanoma of the head and neck. Clin Plast Surg 1976;3:413–27.
7. Carlson GW, Murray DR, Lyles RH, et al. Sentinel lymph node biopsy in the management of cutaneous head and neck melanoma. Plast Reconstr Surg 2005;115:721–8.
8. Green AC, Kimlin M, Siskind V, et al. Hypothesis: hair cover can protect against invasive melanoma on the head and neck (Australia). Cancer Causes Control 2006;17:1263–6.

9. Bodenham DC. Malignant melanoma of head and neck. In: Chambers RD, editor. Cancer of the head and neck. Amsterdam: Excerpta Medica; 1975.

10. Byers RM, Smith JL, Russell N, et al. Malignant melanoma of the external ear. Review of 102 cases. Am J Surg 1980;140:518–21.

11. Bono A, Bartoli C, Maurichi A, et al. Melanoma of the external ear. Tumori 1997; 83:814–7.

12. Breuninger H, Schlagenhauff B, Stroebel W, et al. Patterns of local horizontal spread of melanomas: consequences for surgery and histopathologic investigation. Am J Surg Pathol 1999;23:1493–8.

13. Pack GT, Conley J, Oropeza R. Melanoma of the external ear. Arch Otolaryngol 1970;92:106–13.

14. O'Brien CJ, Coates AS, Petersen-Schaefer K, et al. Experience with 998 cutaneous melanomas of the head and neck over 30 years. Am J Surg 1991;162:310–4.

15. Evans RD, Kopf AW, Lew RA, et al. Risk factors for the development of malignant melanoma–I: Review of case-control studies. J Dermatol Surg Oncol 1988;14:393–408.

16. Chang YM, Barrett JH, Bishop DT, et al. Sun exposure and melanoma risk at different latitudes: a pooled analysis of 5700 cases and 7216 controls. Int J Epidemiol 2009;38:814–30.

17. Caini S, Gandini S, Sera F, et al. Meta-analysis of risk factors for cutaneous melanoma according to anatomical site and clinico-pathological variant. Eur J Cancer 2009;45:3054–63.

18. Elwood JM, Gallagher RP, Hill GB, et al. Pigmentation and skin reaction to sun as risk factors for cutaneous melanoma: Western Canada Melanoma Study. Br Med J (Clin Res Ed) 1984;288:99–102.

19. Kanetaka S, Tsukuda M, Takahashi M, et al. Mucosal melanoma of the head and neck. Exp Ther Med 2011;2:907–10.

20. Younes MN, Myers JN. Melanoma of the head and neck: current concepts in staging, diagnosis, and management. Surg Oncol Clin N Am 2004;13:201–29.

21. Hayward NK. Genetics of melanoma predisposition. Oncogene 2003;22: 3053–62.

22. Gachon J, Beaulieu P, Sei JF, et al. First prospective study of the recognition process of melanoma in dermatological practice. Arch Dermatol 2005;141:434–8.

23. Mackie RM, editor. Illustrated guide to recognition of early malignant melanoma. Edinburgh (United Kingdom): Blackwood, Pillans & Wilson; 1986.

24. Au A, Ariyan S. Melanoma of the head and neck. J Craniofac Surg 2011;22: 421–9.

25. Balch CM, Gershenwald JE, Soong SJ, et al. Final version of 2009 AJCC melanoma staging and classification. J Clin Oncol 2009;27:6199–206.

26. Augenstein AC, Capello ZJ, Little JA, et al. The importance of ulceration of cutaneous melanoma of the head and neck: a comparison of ear (pinna) and nonear sites. Laryngoscope 2012;122:2468–72.

27. McMasters KM. What good is sentinel lymph node biopsy for melanoma if it does not improve survival? Ann Surg Oncol 2004;11:810–2.

28. Prichard RS, Hill AD, Skehan SJ, et al. Positron emission tomography for staging and management of malignant melanoma. Br J Surg 2002;89:389–96.

29. Tyler DS, Onaitis M, Kherani A, et al. Positron emission tomography scanning in malignant melanoma. Cancer 2000;89:1019–25.

30. Bikhchandani J, Wood J, Richards AT, et al. No benefit in staging FDG-PET in cN0 head and neck cutaneous melanoma. Head Neck 2013. http://dx.doi.org/10.1002/hed.23456.

31. Stone M. Initial surgical management of melanoma of the skin and unusual sites. UpToDate; 2013. Available at: http://www.uptodate.com/contents/initial-surgical-management-of-melanoma-of-the-skin-and-unusual-sites.

32. Breslow A, Macht SD. Optimal size of resection margin for thin cutaneous melanoma. Surg Gynecol Obstet 1977;145:691–2.

33. Urist MM, Balch CM, Soong S, et al. The influence of surgical margins and prognostic factors predicting the risk of local recurrence in 3445 patients with primary cutaneous melanoma. Cancer 1985;55:1398–402.

34. Bichakjian CK, Halpern AC, Johnson TM, et al. Guidelines of care for the management of primary cutaneous melanoma. American Academy of Dermatology. J Am Acad Dermatol 2011;65:1032–47.

35. Morton DL, Cochran AJ, Thompson JF, et al. Sentinel node biopsy for early-stage melanoma: accuracy and morbidity in MSLT-I, an international multicenter trial. Ann Surg 2005;242:302–11 [discussion: 311–3].

36. Robinson DS, Sample WF, Fee HJ, et al. Regional lymphatic drainage in primary malignant melanoma of the trunk determined by colloidal gold scanning. Surg Forum 1977;28:147–8.

37. Morton DL, Thompson JF, Essner R, et al. Validation of the accuracy of intraoperative lymphatic mapping and sentinel lymphadenectomy for early-stage melanoma: a multicenter trial. Multicenter Selective Lymphadenectomy Trial Group. Ann Surg 1999;230:453–63 [discussion: 463–5].

38. Rossi CR, De Salvo GL, Trifiro G, et al. The impact of lymphoscintigraphy technique on the outcome of sentinel node biopsy in 1,313 patients with cutaneous melanoma: an Italian Multicentric Study (SOLISM-IMI). J Nucl Med 2006;47:234–41.

39. Testori A, De Salvo GL, Montesco MC, et al. Clinical considerations on sentinel node biopsy in melanoma from an Italian multicentric study on 1,313 patients (SOLISM-IMI). Ann Surg Oncol 2009;16:2018–27.

40. Schmalbach CE, Johnson TM, Bradford CR. The management of head and neck melanoma. In: Flint PW, Haughey BH, Lund VJ, et al, editors. Cummings otolaryngology-head and neck surgery. Philadelphia: Elsevier Mosby; 2005. p. 1115.

41. Leong SP, Accortt NA, Essner R, et al. Impact of sentinel node status and other risk factors on the clinical outcome of head and neck melanoma patients. Arch Otolaryngol Head Neck Surg 2006;132:370–3.

42. Erman AB, Collar RM, Griffith KA, et al. Sentinel lymph node biopsy is accurate and prognostic in head and neck melanoma. Cancer 2012;118:1040–7.

43. Parrett BM, Kashani-Sabet M, Singer MI, et al. Long-term prognosis and significance of the sentinel lymph node in head and neck melanoma. Otolaryngol Head Neck Surg 2012;147(4):699–706.

44. Davis-Malesevich MV, Goepfert R, Kubik M, et al. Recurrence of cutaneous melanoma of the head and neck after negative sentinel lymph node biopsy. Head Neck 2014. http://dx.doi.org/10.1002/hed.23718.

45. Dias Moreira R, Altino de Almeida S, Maliska Guimaraes CM, et al. Sentinel node identification by scintigraphic methods in cutaneous melanoma. J Exp Clin Cancer Res 2005;24:181–5.

46. Tanis PJ, Nieweg OE, van den Brekel MW, et al. Dilemma of clinically node-negative head and neck melanoma: outcome of "watch and wait" policy, elective lymph node dissection, and sentinel node biopsy–a systematic review. Head Neck 2008;30:380–9.

47. Nasri S, Namazie A, Dulguerov P, et al. Malignant melanoma of cervical and parotid lymph nodes with an unknown primary site. Laryngoscope 1994;104:1194–8.

48. Bodem JP, Gulicher D, Engel M, et al. Role of neck dissection in the treatment of melanoma of the head and neck. J Craniofac Surg 2013;24:483–7.
49. O'Brien CJ, Petersen-Schaefer K, Ruark D, et al. Radical, modified, and selective neck dissection for cutaneous malignant melanoma. Head Neck 1995;17: 232–41.
50. Schmalbach CE, Nussenbaum B, Rees RS, et al. Reliability of sentinel lymph node mapping with biopsy for head and neck cutaneous melanoma. Arch Otolaryngol Head Neck Surg 2003;129:61–5.
51. Eicher SA, Clayman GL, Myers JN, et al. A prospective study of intraoperative lymphatic mapping for head and neck cutaneous melanoma. Arch Otolaryngol Head Neck Surg 2002;128:241–6.
52. Suton P, Luksic I, Muller D, et al. Lymphatic drainage patterns of head and neck cutaneous melanoma: does primary melanoma site correlate with anatomic distribution of pathologically involved lymph nodes? Int J Oral Maxillofac Surg 2012;41:413–20.
53. Pathak I, O'Brien CJ, Petersen-Schaeffer K, et al. Do nodal metastases from cutaneous melanoma of the head and neck follow a clinically predictable pattern? Head Neck 2001;23:785–90.
54. Barr LC, Skene AI, Fish S, et al. Superficial parotidectomy in the treatment of cutaneous melanoma of the head and neck. Br J Surg 1994;81:64–5.
55. Samra S, Sawh-Martinez R, Tom L, et al. A targeted approach to sentinel lymph node biopsies in the parotid region for head and neck melanomas. Ann Plast Surg 2012;69:415–7.
56. Ollila DW, Foshag LJ, Essner R, et al. Parotid region lymphatic mapping and sentinel lymphadenectomy for cutaneous melanoma. Ann Surg Oncol 1999;6:150–4.
57. Wells KE, Stadelmann WK, Rapaport DP, et al. Parotid selective lymphadenectomy in malignant melanoma. Ann Plast Surg 1999;43:1–6.
58. Hayashi T, Furukawa H, Oyama A, et al. Dominant lymph drainage in the facial region: evaluation of lymph nodes of facial melanoma patients. Int J Clin Oncol 2012;17:330–5.
59. Peach HS, van der Ploeg AP, Haydu LE, et al. The unpredictability of lymphatic drainage from the ear in melanoma patients, and its implications for management. Ann Surg Oncol 2013;20:1707–13.
60. Gyorki DE, Boyle JO, Ganly I, et al. Incidence and location of positive nonsentinel lymph nodes in head and neck melanoma. Eur J Surg Oncol 2014;40:305–10.
61. Mack LA, McKinnon JG. Controversies in the management of metastatic melanoma to regional lymphatic basins. J Surg Oncol 2004;86:189–99.
62. Shah JP, Kraus DH, Dubner S, et al. Patterns of regional lymph node metastases from cutaneous melanomas of the head and neck. Am J Surg 1991; 162:320–3.
63. Ballo MT, Bonnen MD, Garden AS, et al. Adjuvant irradiation for cervical lymph node metastases from melanoma. Cancer 2003;97:1789–96.
64. Wazer DE. Role of radiation therapy in the management of melanoma. Uptodate; 2013. Available at: http://www.uptodate.com/contents/role-of-radiation-therapy-in-the-management-of-melanoma.
65. Trotti A, Peters LJ. Role of radiotherapy in the primary management of mucosal melanoma of the head and neck. Semin Surg Oncol 1993;9:246–50.
66. Temam S, Mamelle G, Marandas P, et al. Postoperative radiotherapy for primary mucosal melanoma of the head and neck. Cancer 2005;103:313–9.
67. Kingdom TT, Kaplan MJ. Mucosal melanoma of the nasal cavity and paranasal sinuses. Head Neck 1995;17:184–9.

68. Owens JM, Roberts DB, Myers JN. The role of postoperative adjuvant radiation therapy in the treatment of mucosal melanomas of the head and neck region. Arch Otolaryngol Head Neck Surg 2003;129:864–8.

69. Balm AJ, Kroon BB, de Boer JB, et al. Report of a symposium on: diagnosis and treatment of cutaneous head and neck melanoma. Eur J Surg Oncol 1994;20:112–4.

70. Kirkwood JM, Strawderman MH, Ernstoff MS, et al. Interferon alfa-2b adjuvant therapy of high-risk resected cutaneous melanoma: the Eastern Cooperative Oncology Group Trial EST 1684. J Clin Oncol 1996;14:7–17.

71. Creagan ET, Schaid DJ, Ahmann DL, et al. Disseminated malignant melanoma and recombinant interferon: analysis of seven consecutive phase II investigations. J Invest Dermatol 1990;95:188S–92S.

72. Wheatley K, Ives N, Hancock B, et al. Does adjuvant interferon-alpha for high-risk melanoma provide a worthwhile benefit? A meta-analysis of the randomised trials. Cancer Treat Rev 2003;29:241–52.

73. Mocellin S, Pasquali S, Rossi CR, et al. Interferon alpha adjuvant therapy in patients with high-risk melanoma: a systematic review and meta-analysis. J Natl Cancer Inst 2010;102:493–501.

74. Thomas JR, Frost TW. Immediate versus delayed repair of skin defects following resection of carcinoma. Otolaryngol Clin North Am 1993;26:203–13.

75. Escobar V, Zide MF. Delayed repair of skin cancer defects. J Oral Maxillofac Surg 1999;57:271–9 [discussion: 279–80].

76. Bumsted RM, Panje WR, Ceilley RI. Delayed skin grafting in facial reconstruction. When to use and how to do. Arch Otolaryngol 1983;109:178–84.

77. Bogle M, Kelly P, Shenaq J, et al. The role of soft tissue reconstruction after melanoma resection in the head and neck. Head Neck 2001;23:8–15.

78. Sullivan SR, Liu DZ, Mathes DW, et al. Head and neck malignant melanoma: local recurrence rate following wide local excision and immediate reconstruction. Ann Plast Surg 2012;68:33–6.

79. Sullivan SR, Scott JR, Cole JK, et al. Head and neck malignant melanoma: margin status and immediate reconstruction. Ann Plast Surg 2009;62:144–8.

80. van Aalst JA, McCurry T, Wagner J. Reconstructive considerations in the surgical management of melanoma. Surg Clin North Am 2003;83:187–230.

81. Cormack GC, Lamberty BG. Fasciocutaneous vessels in the upper arm: application to the design of new fasciocutaneous flaps. Plast Reconstr Surg 1984;74:244–50.

82. Joss GS, Zoltie N, Chapman P. Tissue expansion technique and the transposition flap. Br J Plast Surg 1990;43:328–33.

83. Khosh MM. Full-thickness skin grafts. Medscape; 2012. Available at: http://emedicine.medscape.com/article/876379-overview.

84. Wax MK, Ghanem TA. Split-thickness skin grafts. Medscape; 2013. Available at: http://emedicine.medscape.com/article/876290-overview.

85. White N, Hettiaratchy S, Papini RP. The choice of split-thickness skin graft donor site: patients' and surgeons' preferences. Plast Reconstr Surg 2003;112:933–4.

86. Sclafan AP. Rhombic flaps. Medscape; 2013. Available at: http://emedicine.medscape.com/article/879923-overview.

87. Lin SJ. Head and neck cancer - reconstruction. Medscape; 2012. Available at: http://emedicine.medscape.com/article/1289799-overview.

88. Mureau MA, Posch NA, Meeuwis CA, et al. Anterolateral thigh flap reconstruction of large external facial skin defects: a follow-up study on functional and aesthetic recipient- and donor-site outcome. Plast Reconstr Surg 2005;115:1077–86.

89. Evans GR, Schusterman MA, Kroll SS, et al. The radial forearm free flap for head and neck reconstruction: a review. Am J Surg 1994;168:446–50.

90. Chalmers RL, Smock E, Geh JL. Experience of Integra(®) in cancer reconstructive surgery. J Plast Reconstr Aesthet Surg 2010;63:2081–90.
91. Moncrieff MD, Spira K, Clark JR, et al. Free flap reconstruction for melanoma of the head and neck: indications and outcomes. J Plast Reconstr Aesthet Surg 2010;63:205–12.
92. Onishi K, Maruyama Y, Hayashi A, et al. Repair of scalp defect using a superficial temporal fascia pedicle VY advancement scalp flap. Br J Plast Surg 2005; 58:676–80.
93. Eshima I. The role of plastic surgery in the treatment of malignant melanoma. Surg Clin North Am 1996;76:1331–42.
94. Jansen L, Koops HS, Nieweg OE, et al. Sentinel node biopsy for melanoma in the head and neck region. Head Neck 2000;22:27–33.
95. Beasley NJ, Gilbert RW, Gullane PJ, et al. Scalp and forehead reconstruction using free revascularized tissue transfer. Arch Facial Plast Surg 2004;6:16–20.
96. McCombe D, Donato R, Hofer SO, et al. Free flaps in the treatment of locally advanced malignancy of the scalp and forehead. Ann Plast Surg 2002;48: 600–6.
97. Mustarde JC. Reconstruction of eyelids. Ann Plast Surg 1983;11:149–69.
98. Spinelli HM, Jelks GW. Periocular reconstruction: a systematic approach. Plast Reconstr Surg 1993;91:1017–24 [discussion: 1025–6].
99. Briele HA, Walker MJ, Das Gupta TK. Melanoma of the head and neck. Clin Plast Surg 1985;12:495–504.
100. Driscoll BP, Baker SR. Reconstruction of nasal alar defects. Arch Facial Plast Surg 2001;3:91–9.
101. Rohrich RJ, Griffin JR, Ansari M, et al. Nasal reconstruction–beyond aesthetic subunits: a 15-year review of 1334 cases. Plast Reconstr Surg 2004;114: 1405–16 [discussion: 1417–9].
102. Park SS. Reconstruction of nasal defects larger than 1.5 centimeters in diameter. Laryngoscope 2000;110:1241–50.
103. Menick FJ. A 10-year experience in nasal reconstruction with the three-stage forehead flap. Plast Reconstr Surg 2002;109:1839–55 [discussion: 1856–61].
104. Pribaz JJ, Falco N. Nasal reconstruction with auricular microvascular transplant. Ann Plast Surg 1993;31:289–97.
105. Ozek C, Gurler T, Uckan A, et al. Reconstruction of the distal third of the nose with composite ear-helix free flap. Ann Plast Surg 2007;58:74–7.
106. Bartell HL, Bedikian AY, Papadopoulos NE, et al. Biochemotherapy in patients with advanced head and neck mucosal melanoma. Head Neck 2008;30:1592–8.
107. Pockaj BA, Jaroszewski DE, DiCaudo DJ, et al. Changing surgical therapy for melanoma of the external ear. Ann Surg Oncol 2003;10:689–96.
108. Narayan D, Ariyan S. Surgical considerations in the management of malignant melanoma of the ear. Plast Reconstr Surg 2001;107:20–4.
109. Antia NH, Buch VI. Chondrocutaneous advancement flap for the marginal defect of the ear. Plast Reconstr Surg 1967;39:472–7.
110. Butler CE. Reconstruction of marginal ear defects with modified chondrocutaneous helical rim advancement flaps. Plast Reconstr Surg 2003;111:2009–13.
111. Katzbach R, Frenzel H, Klaiber S, et al. Borderline indications for ear reconstruction. Ann Plast Surg 2006;57:626–30.
112. Etzkorn JR, Cherpelis BS, Glass LF. Mohs surgery for melanoma: rationale, advances and possibilities. Expert Rev Anticancer Ther 2011;11:1041–52.
113. Hunt JP, Florell SR, Buchmann LO. Rare skin malignancies of the head and neck: a review. Facial Plast Surg 2013;29:389–93.

Melanoma in Non-Caucasian Populations

Jonathan Stubblefield, BS[a], Brent Kelly, MD[b],*

KEYWORDS

- Melanoma • Acral lentiginous melanoma • Non-Caucasians

KEY POINTS

- Melanoma is the most dangerous form of skin cancer.
- Non-Caucasian populations have a higher incidence of the acral lentiginous subtype of melanoma, which is seen on non–sun-exposed areas such as the palms, soles, and subungual sites.
- Darker skin is thought to play a protective role against ultraviolet radiation–induced damage, but the role of melanin is still under investigation.
- Non-Caucasians are more likely to have late-stage disease diagnosed at initial presentation and have higher mortality rates than whites.
- Acral lentiginous melanoma has specific genetic alterations in genes such as KIT, NRAS, and cyclin D1.
- Research investigating better disease education and screening techniques has found promising results for addressing the disparities in melanoma among ethnic groups.

INTRODUCTION

Melanoma is the most dangerous form of skin cancer and the sixth leading cause of malignancy in the United States. Its pathophysiology is not yet completely understood, but fair skin has been identified as a significant risk factor.[1] Melanoma begins as a malignant change in skin melanocytes. The cause of the change is still debated, but ultraviolet (UV) radiation is thought to play a large part in the process. During early stages, the tumor grows contiguously and usually in a radial pattern spreading out along the dermoepidermal junction. Specific genetic alterations occur that shift the tumor's growth from a radial distribution to vertical, which leads to the tumor becoming invasive and eventually metastasizing.[2]

The authors have nothing to disclose.
[a] School of Medicine, University of Texas Medical Branch, 301 University Boulevard, Galveston, TX 77555, USA; [b] Department of Dermatology, University of Texas Medical Branch, 301 University Boulevard, 4.112 McCullough Building, Galveston, TX 77555-0783, USA
* Corresponding author.
E-mail address: bckelly@utmb.edu

Most research on melanoma has focused on Caucasian populations because of the increased incidence in lighter-skinned individuals. For example, a recent study reported a lifetime risk of melanoma of 1 in 52 across all populations. African Americans, however, have a lifetime risk of less than 1 per 1000.[3] Numerous research studies examined the impact of melanoma on African American populations, but the literature on other non-Caucasian ethnic groups is sparse.

African Americans and other ethnic groups often have more advanced disease than Caucasian populations at the time of initial diagnosis. This likely is a major contributor to the higher mortality rate associated with melanoma in more darkly pigmented populations.[4] The advanced disease at presentation is theorized to be caused by the anatomic differences in melanoma location (eg, acral lentiginous), lower socioeconomic status, and education level.[1,5-8]

One factor thought to impact survival in non-Caucasians is poor screening techniques and decreased awareness of differences between whites and non-Caucasians in the presentation of cutaneous melanoma. Promoting increased awareness among patients and health care providers can help reduce the disparity in melanoma outcomes between ethnic groups.

EPIDEMIOLOGY
Anatomy

Anatomically, African Americans and other ethnic groups are more commonly diagnosed with the acral lentiginous subtype of melanoma, which presents on the palms, soles, and subungual sites.[4,5] When compared with Caucasians, this may pose a challenge for both patient and provider when it comes to noticing early disease. For instance, one study examined data from the Surveillance, Epidemiology, and End Results (SEER) database and found an overall lower incidence of melanoma among Hispanics, African Americans, American Indians, and Asians but a higher proportion of lower-extremity lesions and acral lentiginous melanoma.[9] In a study examining a cohort of 1439 black patients, the lower limbs were found to be the most common site of melanoma.[10]

Hemmings and colleagues[4] compared whites with nonwhites and found a significantly higher incidence of melanoma on the sole and subungual locations in nonwhite populations. The same study reported a decreased incidence of melanoma in the typical sun-exposed areas such as head, neck, and trunk in nonwhites. This atypical distribution may contribute to disparities in disease detection and lead to later stages of disease at diagnosis in non-Caucasians.[4,11] Education and improved screening techniques may reduce differences in melanoma outcomes in darker-skinned populations.

Clinical Presentation

Acral lentiginous melanoma lesions are often initially clinically misdiagnosed as more benign diseases (**Fig. 1**). Soon and colleagues[12] reported that up to one-half are diagnosed as warts, ulcers, hematomas, foreign bodies, or fungal infections. For example, Ise and colleagues[13] reported a case in Japan of an acral melanoma on the sole with hyperkeratosis that mimicked a pigmented wart in appearance. Dysplastic nevi are intermediate lesions between regular nevi and melanoma. Differentiating dysplastic nevi from melanoma remains a challenge for providers, but Argenziano and colleagues[14] found dermoscopy to be a valid method for differentiating dysplastic nevi from melanoma. Melanonychia is a condition in which nail bed melanocytes become activated and cause the nail to appear black or brown. It is often

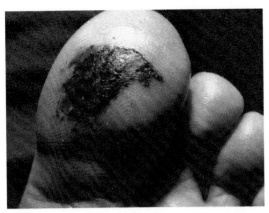

Fig. 1. An acral lentiginous melanoma on the great toe of a middle-aged Latin American woman. The lesion had been treated for months as a chronic wound.

seen as a hyperpigmented longitudinal band on the nail (**Fig. 2**).[15] Approximately two-thirds of melanomas in the nail area can present with melanonychia,[16] but melanonychia can also be a manifestation of many benign conditions, such as trauma or onychomycosis.[15] Acral melanoma can also present as a chronic wound. Yin and colleagues[17] stressed the importance of biopsy in diagnosis after describing a case of a chronic, nonhealing ulcer on the plantar surface of the foot that revealed acral melanoma when biopsied.

Histologic Type

Acral lentiginous melanoma is the fourth most common form of malignant melanoma and makes up a very small proportion of all histologic subtypes. It is characterized by an acral distribution of lesions, meaning that neoplasms are seen on the extremities. The word *lentiginous* refers to the radial growth phase when the tumor is confined to tissue above the basement membrane. Histologically, acral melanoma consists of confluent dendritic melanocytes, both singly and in nests along the dermal-epidermal junction with varying amounts of upward pagetoid migration (**Figs. 3** and **4**). Extension

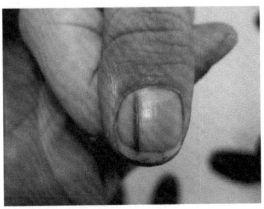

Fig. 2. Melanonychia. This lesion was found to be benign. Hutchinson's sign is not present.

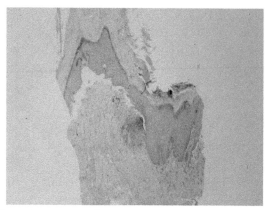

Fig. 3. Hematoxylin and eosin stain (20×) shows acral skin with artifactual subepidermal split.

down adnexal structures is common. The individual cells in the epidermis are often dendritic but can be epithelioid as well. Nuclear atypia, pleomorphism, and hyperchromasia are apparent. The pagetoid or ascending cells often extend into the stratum corneum. The surrounding epidermis is often thickened (as opposed to lentigo maligna melanoma where it is atrophic). Dermal invasion is often in the form of atypical epithelioid nests or cords. Occasionally, the dermal component is spindled and can show a desmoplastic appearance. Lymphocytic inflammation and intermittent areas of fibrosis are often seen. Ulceration, regression, and deep extension are other worrisome features that may be present. Subungual melanomas may have a similar histologic subtype but often are histologically similar to the superficial spreading melanoma subtype. Adequate biopsy specimens are critical, particularly for subungual lesions, which may be technically difficult. Another histologic pitfall in the interpretation of subungual lesions is that melanocytes in normal nail matrix can have a pagetoid appearance.[18] Subungual melanoma poses a unique challenge to providers because of the need to biopsy the lesions. Numerous methods for taking samples of nail matrix tissue exist; however, if suspicion

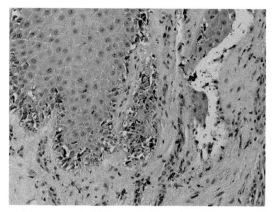

Fig. 4. Hematoxylin and eosin stain (400×). Higher power shows marked atypia of melanocytes in the basal layer that are contiguous and stacked. The cells are dyscohesive, and pigment incontinence is prominent.

for invasive melanoma is high, full-thickness excisional biopsy is recommended.[19] To take an adequate sample from the nail matrix, the nail must often be removed, and a large elliptical incision is made over the nail bed under local or regional anesthesia. Tissue is removed down to the periosteum, and the wound is then closed. Providers must have strong clinical suspicion for melanoma rather than a more benign condition, such as a subungual hematoma, before performing a biopsy or excision because of the deforming nature of the procedure.

In non-Caucasian populations, the incidence of the acral lentiginous subtype is higher than in Caucasians.[4,6,9,20] One study reported that it accounted for 58% of melanomas in Asians,[21] and another reported that it comprised 60% to 70% of melanomas in African Americans.[22] The subungual subtype of acral lentiginous melanoma is even rarer, making up 0.7% to .5% of melanomas across all populations, but it makes up as much as 75% of cases in non-Caucasian populations.[23,24] The histopathologic subtype of acral lentiginous melanoma does not itself affect prognosis, but the higher mortality rate associated with this type is believed to be attributed to the atypical distribution of lesions that affect the likelihood of early diagnosis.[4,5]

Stage at Diagnosis

Numerous studies document that African Americans and other non-Caucasian groups present with late-stage disease and that stage at diagnosis is a strong predictor of survival. Poor access to health care as a result of lower socioeconomic status may be associated with more advanced disease.[7,8] One study examined melanoma specifically in the African American population over 2 decades and found that Caucasians were 3.6 times more likely to have early-stage disease diagnosed compared with blacks. This finding led to a difference in survival time between Caucasians and African Americans.[6] Hemmings and colleagues[4] reported that nonwhite patients were more likely to have thicker tumors at initial diagnosis and were also more likely to have ulcerated lesions in a study involving 357 patients. Ulcerated lesions are strongly associated with poorer prognosis compared with nonulcerated lesions, and the presence of ulceration is routinely included when staging melanomas.[25]

Another study conducted from 1988 to 2001 reported an 11.6% increase in the number of Hispanic men presenting with tumors thicker than 1.5 mm compared with a 1.8% increase in overall melanoma incidence, showing a disproportionate increase in the amount of advanced disease.[26] A study examining the incidence of melanoma in California Hispanics found a statistically significant higher rate of increased tumor thickness at diagnosis in Hispanics despite a higher overall incidence of melanoma in non-Hispanic whites.[7] Park and colleagues[1] studied a large cohort of 101,229 non-Caucasians that covered numerous ethnic groups including Asians, Hispanics, African Americans, Pacific Islanders, and multiethnic people. They found a statistically significantly higher risk for nonwhite women to have a diagnosis of late-stage disease.

Non-Caucasians are also more likely to have disease that has spread to lymph nodes or have distant metastasis at initial diagnosis. Hemmings and colleagues[4] reported that nonwhite patients were more likely to have nodal spread and an advanced stage when melanoma is initially diagnosed. Byrd and colleagues[11] reported that African American patients were almost 3 times more likely to have stage III or IV melanoma on initial presentation and had a deeper Breslow depth than Caucasians (2.75 mm vs 1.16 mm, respectively). Similarly, another retrospective study of melanoma cases in Florida over a 5-year period reported that Hispanic and black patients were more likely to have regional or distant metastasis of cancer at diagnosis.[27] Another study examining the population in Florida reported similar trends and also noted that although the proportion of late stage- melanomas diagnosed in Caucasians decreased from 1990 to 2004, the amount of late-stage disease diagnosed in Hispanics and blacks stayed the same.[28] A study examining a decade of data from the SEER database reported odds ratios of 4.2, 3.6, 3.4, and 2.4 for African Americans, Hispanics, American Indians, and Asians, respectively, to be diagnosed with stage IV disease.[9]

ETIOLOGY

The etiology of melanoma is a topic of research and debate. Sun exposure has been identified as a strong risk factor in white populations, as evidenced by the higher incidence of lesions in sun-exposed areas on Caucasians.[2,4] In non-Caucasian populations, evidence for specific risk factors has been controversial. Several specific risk factors such as older age, male gender, and lighter-skinned phenotypes for non-Caucasian/non–African American groups have been identified,[1] but the roles of traditionally accepted factors such as sun exposure are still under scrutiny.

Subtype

As previously discussed, African American and other non-Caucasian populations tend to present with the acral lentiginous subtype of melanoma.[4,11] The increased mortality associated with this subtype is often attributed to the fact that patients present at later stages of the disease because the lesions are in less-noticeable areas than other types of melanoma. One study examined a cohort of 126 patients with histologically proven acral lentiginous melanoma to understand the epidemiologic and prognostic factors associated with the specific subtype. That group found no significant relation between overexposure to UV radiation and the incidence of the acral lentiginous subtype of melanoma. Interestingly, the investigators also found no correlation between the incidence of acral melanoma and any genetic traits.[5] This research raises the question of whether groups with pigmented skin have a higher incidence of acral lentiginous melanoma because of a genetic predisposition or if they have relatively higher incidence than Caucasian populations because of a decreased incidence of other subtypes. Further studies are needed to elucidate the role of genetics in acral lentiginous melanoma and to identify specific risk factors associated with this subtype.

UV Radiation

The role of UV radiation is generally accepted as a risk factor for melanoma in fair-skinned populations. Its role in pathogenesis has been extensively researched. For example, one group examined the role of sun exposure in melanoma and found that intermittent sun exposure showed a significantly positive association with the incidence of melanoma, whereas chronic sun exposure showed a significantly reduced risk. The same study found that sunburns also increase the risk of melanoma.[29] Further, researchers have found that only UV B wavelengths initiated melanoma in a mouse model and that mice irradiated with UV A wavelengths even at high doses responded like control groups.[30]

In African American and other non-Caucasian populations, the role of UV radiation in the etiology of melanoma is less clear, and studies are sometimes contradictory. For instance, one study examined the effects of skin melanin content on UV-induced DNA damage after each subject received one minimal erythema dose (MED) of UV radiation. Darker skinned subjects were found to have significantly less DNA damage despite markedly higher UV radiation requirements for one MED. The study also found that only dark-skinned individuals showed substantial increases in melanin content after initial UV exposure. No correlation was found between skin pigment or race and the rate of DNA repair after irradiation.[31] This research suggests a protective role of melanin density against DNA damage and melanoma pathogenesis in non-Caucasian populations.

In contrast, Sheehan and colleagues[32] examined a cohort of patients with Fitzpatrick skin types II and IV and found that physical dose determines the amount of DNA damage. Skin types are classified from I to VI based on their proclivity to burn versus tan, with type I describing fair complexions and type VI referring to black skin. Individuals with darker skin types were found to have more thymine dimers after repeated exposure to 0.65 MED than lighter-skinned individuals exposed to the same fraction of their minimal erythema dose, suggesting a higher rate of DNA damage in dark skin compared with light skin. This finding suggests that melanin does not offer increased protection against DNA damage for darker-skinned populations. This study also found that those with darker skin types showed a significantly increased rate of DNA repair when compared with light-skinned patients. Clearly, current research into disease pathogenesis in non-Caucasians is insufficient, and further research is needed to determine the true role of UV radiation in melanoma pathogenesis in non-Caucasians and to investigate any benefit darker skin types may have for DNA damage repair.

Several studies have attempted to correlate the rates of melanoma in non-Caucasian populations with geographic locations that have higher sun exposure and found various results. Eide and Weinstock[33] examined data from SEER over a decade and divided the patients into blacks, Hispanics, Asian/Pacific Islanders, whites, and Native Americans. They researched the correlation between UV index, latitude, and the incidence of melanoma. The only significant association found between UV exposure and melanoma was in white populations. No correlation between UV index or latitude on melanoma was found in any of the ethnic cohorts. This finding suggests a different mechanism contributing to the incidence of melanoma in dark-skinned people rather than the traditional theory of UV exposure causing DNA damage. However, Hu and colleagues[34] conducted similar research using state cancer registries and found that melanoma incidence was associated with UV index and latitude in Hispanics and blacks. Hu and colleagues'[34] research suggests that UV radiation does contribute to melanoma pathogenesis. Further research is needed to fully understand the role of UV light in the etiology of melanoma.

Genetics

Understanding the specific genetic pathogenesis of melanoma in non-Caucasians will help develop targeted prevention strategies and therapies. As previously discussed, the traditional role of UV light in disease pathogenesis in pigmented skin is still under investigation, and a genetic component may play a role as well. African Americans and other dark-skinned groups have a higher percentage of acral lentiginous melanoma, and this subtype carries some specific genetic mutations.

Several studies have examined the genetic expression of KIT, a tyrosine kinase receptor, in acral and mucosal melanomas. These investigators found increased expression of KIT in these melanoma subtypes suggesting that it plays an important role in disease pathogenesis. This also opens up the possibility of treatment with tyrosine kinase inhibitors such as imatinib (Gleevec).[35,36] Similarly, mutations of BRAF, a gene involved in cell proliferation, have been found to be more common in intermittently sun-damaged skin than chronically sun-damaged skin.[37] This finding correlates with the clinical finding that sunburns and intermittent sun exposure are significant risk factors for melanoma, whereas chronic sun exposure showed a decreased risk. In acral lentiginous melanoma, however, Saldanha and colleagues[38] found a decreased expression of BRAF relative to superficial spreading melanoma, nodular melanoma, and lentigo maligna. Akslen and colleagues[39] found similar results, reporting that blacks had a low percentage of BRAF mutations, which suggests a different pathogenesis in this population. These results support the observation that traditional risk factors such as sunlight are not as important in non-Caucasian melanoma. Understanding the role of BRAF in non-Caucasian disease is critical to optimize the use of BRAF inhibitors such as vemurafenib (Zelboraf) and to develop further targeted strategies for cancer treatment.

Sauter and colleagues[40] examined the expression of cyclin D1, a protein involved in moving through the G1/S checkpoint, in 137 cutaneous melanomas. Using fluorescent in situ hybridization and immunohistochemistry, they found amplification and overexpression of the cyclin D1 gene in 44.4% of acral melanomas compared with 10.5% and 5.6% in lentigo maligna and superficial spreading melanomas, respectively. The same study also examined the role of cyclin D1 in tumor pathogenesis. Downregulation of the cyclin D1 gene in mice by targeted antisense led to significant shrinkage of melanoma tumors, but the growth of normal melanocytes was not affected. This study suggests that overexpression of cyclin D1 may contribute specifically to acral melanoma pathogenesis and that targeted therapies directed at this gene may be an effective form of treatment. Similarly, Ibrahim and colleagues[41] used immunohistochemistry and reported that 68% of acral melanomas positively stained for cyclin D1 expression compared with 33% of nonacral tumors in a retrospective study from 2004 to 2010.

OUTCOMES

Melanoma is the deadliest form of skin cancer and accounts for roughly 75% of deaths from cutaneous malignancies.[42] As previously mentioned, despite a higher awareness of melanoma and its risks, the number of cases of late-stage disease has either increased or stayed relatively constant in non-Caucasian populations while decreasing for whites.[28] This finding has contributed to not only a disparity in the incidence of disease but a disparity of outcomes as well. Blacks and other ethnic groups are at a higher risk of mortality from cutaneous melanoma despite treatment efforts.[42]

Several specific risk factors have been identified for melanomas that are independent predictors of mortality among all populations. For example, Balch and colleagues[25] examined 17,600 melanoma patients to identify specific factors that influenced survival. They subdivided their risk factors according to the tumor-node-metastasis (TNM) staging system and investigated factors affecting each category. Their analysis showed that tumor thickness and the presence of ulceration had the most significant impact on survival within the tumor category, with thickness being a more powerful predictor. Interestingly, the level of invasion was a more important predictor of survival than ulceration in patients with tumors less than 1 mm in thickness. In the node category, the actual number of nodal metastases was the best predictor for survival, with a roughly 50% 5-year survival rate for patients having 1 or 2 nodes positive and a 30% to 40% 5-year survival rate for patients having 3 or more positive nodes. Five-year survival was also impacted by the presence of macroscopic (palpable) versus microscopic nodal disease and primary tumor ulceration. For metastatic disease, the presence of visceral metastasis carried a significantly worse prognosis when compared with patients with metastasis to other skin sites, subcutaneous tissue, or lymph nodes.

Late-stage diagnosis is more common among non-Caucasians than whites, and clearly advanced disease leads to significantly decreased survival times. Bellows and colleagues[6] found that African Americans were more likely to present with late-stage disease, and this led to a median survival time of 90 months less than that of Caucasians (35 vs 145 months). Hemmings and colleagues[4] compared survival rates of white and nonwhite patients using Kaplan-Meier curves and found that nonwhite patients had a decreased overall survival rate, but the disparity between the 2 groups disappeared when the results were stratified by initial stage at diagnosis. This strongly suggests that the increased mortality of non-Caucasian populations is caused by the advanced presentation of disease at diagnosis.

INTERVENTIONS

Increased awareness and screening to catch disease early may help reduce the disparity in outcomes between whites and non-Caucasians. In the general population, Aitken and colleagues[43] studied interventions such as encouraging physician visits, education about self-examinations for skin cancer, and education about when to seek professional medical attention. The intervention group was also provided access to free skin clinics. The authors found that the intervention group showed an increase in the prevalence of physician screenings by as much as 23% above baseline 2 years after starting the intervention. This trend continued, and the intervention group still showed an increase in physician screenings of 8% above baseline 5 years after the study once the access to free skin clinics was removed. Kundu and colleagues[44] studied a cohort of Asian, African American, and Hispanic patients. They examined the impact of education about the "ABCDE" method (asymmetry, border irregularity, color variegation, and diameter) of screening and education about melanoma itself. After the intervention, knowledge that melanoma is a form of skin cancer and knowledge of the risk of melanoma in ethnic groups increased by 16% and 34%, respectively. Similarly, 85% of study participants reported checking acral locations for skin cancer after the intervention compared with 18.7% before the study. This difference remained statistically significant at 3 months, with 67.6% of participants still reporting that they performed self-examinations on acral areas.

Robinson and colleagues[45] examined a group consisting of African Americans, Hispanics, and Asians and found that many people in the study group did not believe they were able to get skin cancer. They also did not think that melanoma was a skin cancer or a relevant concern. The subjects were shown a picture of acral lentiginous melanoma on a subungual site, and many reported that they did not know they could get skin cancer in non–sun-exposed sites, but they reported that seeing the picture made them more likely to perform self-examinations.

Despite treatment efforts, non-Caucasians have higher mortality rates than whites. Byrd and colleagues[11] reported a 5-year survival rate of 58.8% in African Americans compared with 84.8% in whites in a group of 649 patients. Collins and colleagues[42] studied 151,154 patients with primary melanoma and found that 10-year survival rates were lowest in blacks (73%) when compared with whites (88%) and other races (85%). The study also reported that blacks that underwent biopsy, wide excision, or surgery had a significantly reduced mortality rate than whites that underwent the same treatment. However, there was no difference in survival rates between whites and blacks who did not have surgical treatment. This raises questions about possible differences in disease processes between races that might affect treatment outcomes. More research is needed to further clarify the best treatment option for African Americans and other dark-skinned populations.

SUMMARY

Clinical presentation may be a large contributing factor to the disparity in outcomes between light- and dark-skinned populations with melanoma. The atypical distribution of melanoma lesions on pigmented skin may delay detection and lead to a higher incidence of late-stage diagnosis than Caucasian populations.[4,11,27,28] As previously discussed, studies that have examined the effects of raising awareness and promoting screening have shown promising results.[43–45] Raising awareness about the distributions of lesions in non-Caucasian populations can prevent late-stage diagnosis and help reduce mortality rates from melanoma in this cohort. Education is critical to teach both patients and physicians to check for lesions in sun-protected areas. Establishing specific screening methods may help reduce the mortality of melanoma in non-Caucasian populations. Techniques such as the ABCD method first mentioned by Friedman and colleagues[46] for detecting melanoma in which providers or patients check skin lesions for asymmetry, border irregularity, color variegation, and evaluate a lesion's diameter provide useful screening tools that can be used to improve detection of early disease in non-Caucasian populations.

REFERENCES

1. Park S, Marchand L, Wilkens L, et al. Risk factors for malignant melanoma in white and non-white/Non-African American populations; the multiethnic cohort. Cancer Prev Res (Phila) 2012;5:423–34.
2. Alexandrescu D, Maslin B, Kauffman C, et al. Malignant melanoma in pigmented skin: does the current interventional model fit a different clinical, histologic, and molecular entity? Dematol Surg 2013;39:1291–303.
3. Altekruse SF, Kosary CL, Krapcho M, et al, editors. SEER cancer statistics review, 1975–2007. Bethesda (MD): National Cancer Institute; 2010. based on November 2009 SEER data submission, posted to the SEER web site. Available at: http://seer.cancer.gov/csr/1975_2007/.
4. Hemmings DE, Johnson DS, Tominaga GT, et al. Cutaneous melanoma in a multiethnic population: is this a different disease? Arch Surg 2004;139:968–72 [discussion: 972–3].
5. Phan A, Touzet S, Dalle S, et al. Acral lentiginous melanoma: a clinicoprognostic study of 126 cases. Br J Dermatol 2006;155:561–9.
6. Bellows CF, Belafsky P, Fortgang IS, et al. Melanoma in African-Americans: trends in biological behavior and clinical characteristics over two decades. J Surg Oncol 2001;78:10–6.
7. Pollitt R, Clarke C, Swetter S, et al. The expanding melanoma burden in california hispanics. Cancer 2011;117:152–61.
8. Zell J, Cinar P, Mobasher M, et al. Survival for patients with invasive cutaneous melanoma among Ethnic Groups: the effects of socioeconomic status and treatment. J Clin Oncol 2008;26:66–75.
9. Cormier JN, Xing Y, Ding M, et al. Ethnic differences among patients with cutaneous melanoma. Arch Intern Med 2006;166:1907–14.
10. Myles Z, Buchanan N, King J, et al. Anatomic distribution of malignant melanoma on the non-hispanic black patient, 1998-2007. Arch Dermatol 2012;148:797–801.
11. Byrd KM, Wilson DC, Hoyler SS, et al. Advanced presentation of melanoma in African Americans. J Am Acad Dermatol 2004;50:21–4.
12. Soon SL, Solomon AR Jr, Papadopoulos D, et al. Acral lentiginous melanoma mimicking benign disease: the Emory experience. J Am Acad Dermatol 2003; 48:183–8.

13. Ise M, Yasuda F, Konohana I, et al. Acral melanoma with hyperkeratosis mimicking a pigmented wart. Dermatol Pract Concept 2013;3:37–9.
14. Argenziano G, Soyer HP, Chimenti S, et al. Dermoscopy of pigmented skin lesions: results of a consensus meeting via the Internet. J Am Acad Dermatol 2003;48:679–93.
15. Andre J, Lateur N. Pigmented nail disorders. Dermatol Clin 2006;24(3):329–39.
16. Haneke E, Baran R. Longitudinal melanonychia. Dermatol Surg 2001;27(6): 580–4.
17. Yin N, Miteva M, Covington D, et al. The importance of wound biopsy in the accurate diagnosis of acral malignant melanoma presenting as a foot ulcer. Int J Low Extrem Wounds 2013;12:289–92.
18. Perrin C, Michiels J, Pisani A, et al. Anatomic distribution of melanocytes in normal nail unit: an immunohistochemical investigation. Am J Dermatopathol 1997;19:462–7.
19. Jellinek N. Nail matrix biopsy of longitudinal melanonychia: Diagnostic algorithm including the matrix shave biopsy. Dermatol Surg 2007;56:803–10.
20. Stevens NG, Liff JM, Weiss NS. Plantar melanoma: is the incidence of melanoma of the sole of the foot really higher in blacks than whites? Int J Cancer 1990;45: 691–3.
21. Chang J, Yeh K, Wang C. Malignant melanoma in taiwan: a prognostic study of 181 cases. Melanoma Res 2004;14:537–41.
22. Hudson D, Krige J. Melanoma in black south Africans. J Am Coll Surg 1995;180: 65–71.
23. De Giorgi V, Saggini A, Grazzini M, et al. Specific challenges in the management of subungual melanoma. Expert Rev Anticancer Ther 2011;11:749–61.
24. Patel G, Ragi G, Krysicki J, et al. Subungual melanoma: a deceptive disorder. Acta Dermatovenerol Croat 2008;16:236–42.
25. Balch CM, Soong SJ, Gershenwald JE, et al. Prognostic factors analysis of 17,600 melanoma patients: validation of the American Joint Committee on Cancer melanoma staging system. J Clin Oncol 2001;19:3622–34.
26. Cockburn MG, Zadnick J, Deapen D. Developing epidemic of melanoma in the hispanic population of California. Cancer 2006;106:1162–8.
27. Hu S, Soza-Vento R, Parker D, et al. Comparison of stage at diagnosis of melanoma among hispanic, black, and white patients in Miami-Dade County, Florida. Arch Dermatol 2006;142:704–8.
28. Hu S, Parmet Y, Allen G, et al. Disparity in melanoma. Arch Dermatol 2009;145: 1369–74.
29. Elwood JM, Jopson J. Melanoma and sun exposure: an overview of published studies. Int J Cancer 1997;73:198–203.
30. Fabo E, Noonan F, Fears T, et al. Ultraviolet B but not ultraviolet A radiation initiates melanoma. Cancer Res 2004;64:6372–6.
31. Tadokoro T, Kobayashi N, Zmudzka BZ, et al. UV-induced DNA damage and melanin content in human skin differing in racial/ethnic origin. FASEB J 2003; 17:1177–9.
32. Sheehan J, Cragg N, Chadwick C, et al. Repeated ultraviolet exposure affords the same protection against DNAN photodamage and erythema in human skin types II and IV but is associated with faster DNA repair in skin type IV. J Invest Dermatol 2002;118:825–9.
33. Eide MJ, Weinstock MA. Association of UV index, latitude, and melanoma incidence in nonwhite populations—US Surveillance, Epidemiology, and End Results (SEER) Program, 1992 to 2001. Arch Dermatol 2005;141:477–81.

34. Hu S, Ma F, Collado-Mesa F, et al. UV radiation, latitude, and melanoma in US Hispanics and blacks. Arch Dermatol 2004;140:819–24.
35. Curtin JA, Busam K, Pinkel D, et al. Somatic activation of KIT in distinct subtypes of melanoma. J Clin Oncol 2006;24:4340–6.
36. Ashida A, Takata M, Murata H, et al. Pathological activation of KIT in metastatic tumors of acral and mucosal melanomas. Int J Cancer 2009;124:862–8.
37. Curtin JA, Fridlyand J, Kageshita T, et al. Distinct sets of genetic alterations in melanoma. N Engl J Med 2005;353:2135–47.
38. Saldanha G, Potter L, DaForno P, et al. Cutaneous melanoma subtypes show different BRAF and NRAS mutation frequencies. Clin Cancer Res 2006;12: 4499–505.
39. Akslen LA, Puntervoll H, Bachmann IM, et al. Mutation analysis of the EGFR-NRAS-BRAF pathway in melanomas from black Africans and other subgroups of cutaneous melanoma. Melanoma Res 2008;18:29–35.
40. Sauter E, Yeo UC, von Stemm A, et al. Cyclin D1 is a candidate oncogene in cutaneous melanoma. Cancer Res 2002;62:3200–6.
41. Ibrahim Z, Narihan M, Ojep D, et al. Cyclin D1 expression in acral melanoma: a case control study in Sarawak. Malays J Pathol 2012;34:89–95.
42. Collins K, Fields R, Baptiste D, et al. Racial differences in survival after surgical treatment for melanoma. Ann Surg Oncol 2011;18:2925–36.
43. Aitken JF, Youl PH, Janda M, et al. Increase in skin cancer screening during a community-based randomized intervention trial. Int J Cancer 2006;118:1010–6.
44. Kundu R, Kamaria M, Ortiz S, et al. Effectiveness of a knowledge-based intervention for melanoma among those with ethnic skin. J Am Acad Dermatol 2010;62: 777–84.
45. Robinson JK, Joshi KM, Ortiz S, et al. Melanoma knowledge, perception, and awareness in ethnic minorities in Chicago: recommendations regarding education. Psychooncology 2011;20:313–20.
46. Friedman RJ, Rigel DS, Kopf AW. Early detection of malignant melanoma: the role of physician examination and self- examination of the skin. CA Cancer J Clin 1985;35:130–51.

Index

Note: Page numbers of article titles are in **boldface** type.

A

Age
 as factor in melanoma, 947–948
Anorectal melanoma
 RT for, 1035

B

Bacille Calmette-Guerin (BCG)
 in melanoma, 1008
BCG. *See* Bacille Calmette-Guerin (BCG)
BRAF-mutant melanoma
 algorithm for, 1052–1053

C

Chemotherapy
 for HNM, 1100
Chest x-ray
 in workup and staging of malignant melanoma, 967
Children
 cutaneous melanoma arising in, 1064–1065
Cutaneous melanoma
 arising in childhood, 1064–1065
 high-risk
  RT for, 1032–1033
 surviving, **989–1002**. *See also* Melanoma

D

Dermis
 unknown primary melanoma in, 1062–1063
Desmoplastic melanoma
 RT for, 1033

E

Elective lymphadenectomy
 in regional lymph node management, 977–978
Eye(s)
 melanoma arising on, 1067–1069

Surg Clin N Am 94 (2014) 1127–1134
http://dx.doi.org/10.1016/S0039-6109(14)00131-5
0039-6109/14/$ – see front matter © 2014 Elsevier Inc. All rights reserved.

surgical.theclinics.com

United States Postal Service

Statement of Ownership, Management, and Circulation
(All Periodicals Publications Except Requestor Publications)

1. Publication Title	2. Publication Number	3. Filing Date
Surgical Clinics of North America	5 2 9 - 8 0 0 0	9/14/14

4. Issue Frequency	5. Number of Issues Published Annually	6. Annual Subscription Price
Feb, Apr, Jun, Aug, Oct, Dec	6	$370.00

7. Complete Mailing Address of Known Office of Publication (Not printer) (Street, city, county, state, and ZIP+4®)

Elsevier Inc.
360 Park Avenue South
New York, NY 10010-1710

Contact Person
Stephen R. Bushing
Telephone (Include area code)
215-239-3688

8. Complete Mailing Address of Headquarters or General Business Office of Publisher (Not printer)

Elsevier Inc., 360 Park Avenue South, New York, NY 10010-1710

9. Full Names and Complete Mailing Addresses of Publisher, Editor, and Managing Editor (Do not leave blank)

Publisher (Name and complete mailing address)

Linda Belfus, Elsevier, Inc., 1600 John F. Kennedy Blvd. Suite 1800, Philadelphia, PA 19103-2899

Editor (Name and complete mailing address)

John Vassallo, Elsevier, Inc. 1600 John F. Kennedy Blvd. Suite 1800, Philadelphia, PA 19103-2899

Managing Editor (Name and complete mailing address)

Adrianne Brigido, Elsevier, Inc., 1600 John F. Kennedy Blvd. Suite 1800, Philadelphia, PA 19103-2899

10. Owner (Do not leave blank. If the publication is owned by a corporation, give the name and address of the corporation immediately followed by the names and addresses of all stockholders owning or holding 1 percent or more of the total amount of stock. If not owned by a corporation, give the names and addresses of the individual owners. If owned by a partnership or other unincorporated firm, give its name and address as well as those of each individual owner. If the publication is published by a nonprofit organization, give its name and address.)

Full Name	Complete Mailing Address
Wholly owned subsidiary of	1600 John F. Kennedy Blvd, Ste. 1800
Reed/Elsevier, US holdings	Philadelphia, PA 19103-2899

11. Known Bondholders, Mortgagees, and Other Security Holders Owning or Holding 1 Percent or More of Total Amount of Bonds, Mortgages, or Other Securities. If none, check box ☑ None

Full Name	Complete Mailing Address
N/A	

12. Tax Status (For completion by nonprofit organizations authorized to mail at nonprofit rates) (Check one)
The purpose, function, and nonprofit status of this organization and the exempt status for federal income tax purposes:
☐ Has Not Changed During Preceding 12 Months
☐ Has Changed During Preceding 12 Months (Publisher must submit explanation of change with this statement)

PS Form 3526, August 2012 (Page 1 of 3 (Instructions Page 3)) PSN 7530-01-000-9931 **PRIVACY NOTICE:** See our Privacy policy in www.usps.com

---

13. Publication Title			14. Issue Date for Circulation Data Below
Surgical Clinics of North America			June 2014

15. Extent and Nature of Circulation			Average No. Copies Each Issue During Preceding 12 Months	No. Copies of Single Issue Published Nearest to Filing Date
a. Total Number of Copies (Net press run)			2,036	2,161
b. Paid Circulation (By Mail and Outside the Mail)	(1)	Mailed Outside-County Paid Subscriptions Stated on PS Form 3541. (Include paid distribution above nominal rate, advertiser's proof copies, and exchange copies)	986	1,071
	(2)	Mailed In-County Paid Subscriptions Stated on PS Form 3541 (Include paid distribution above nominal rate, advertiser's proof copies, and exchange copies)		
	(3)	Paid Distribution Outside the Mails Including Sales Through Dealers and Carriers, Street Vendors, Counter Sales, and Other Paid Distribution Outside USPS®	492	488
	(4)	Paid Distribution by Other Classes Mailed Through the USPS (e.g. First-Class Mail®)		
c. Total Paid Distribution (Sum of 15b (1), (2), (3), and (4))		▶	1,478	1,559
d. Free or Nominal Rate Distribution (By Mail and Outside the Mail)	(1)	Free or Nominal Rate Outside-County Copies Included on PS Form 3541	52	62
	(2)	Free or Nominal Rate In-County Copies Included on PS Form 3541		
	(3)	Free or Nominal Rate Copies Mailed at Other Classes Through the USPS (e.g. First-Class Mail)		
	(4)	Free or Nominal Rate Distribution Outside the Mail (Carriers or other means)		
e. Total Free or Nominal Rate Distribution (Sum of 15d (1), (2), (3) and (4)		▶	52	62
f. Total Distribution (Sum of 15c and 15e)		▶	1,530	1,621
g. Copies not Distributed (See instructions to publishers #4 (page #3))		▶	506	540
h. Total (Sum of 15f and g)		▶	2,036	2,161
i. Percent Paid (15c divided by 15f times 100)		▶	96.60%	96.18%

16. Total circulation includes electronic copies. Report circulation on PS Form 3526-X worksheet.

17. Publication of Statement of Ownership
If the publication is a general publication, publication of this statement is required. Will be printed in the October 2014 issue of this publication.

18. Signature and Title of Editor, Publisher, Business Manager, or Owner	Date
Stephen R. Bushing – Inventory Distribution Coordinator *(signature)*	September 14, 2014

I certify that all information furnished on this form is true and complete. I understand that anyone who furnishes false or misleading information on this form or who omits material or information requested on the form may be subject to criminal sanctions (including fines and imprisonment) and/or civil sanctions (including civil penalties).

PS Form 3526, August 2012 (Page 2 of 3)

Printed and bound by CPI Group (UK) Ltd, Croydon, CR0 4YY

07/10/2024

01040498-0019